AF822553

PHYSEO

TABLE OF CONTENTS

We would like to extend a special thanks to the following individuals who have spent many hours tutoring, guiding and consulting this work, making Physeo Embryology possible.

Paloma F Cariello, MD, MPH
Assistant Professor
Division of Infectious Diseases
University of Utah School of Medicine
Salt Lake City, UT

Karen Eilbeck, Ph.D.
Professor
Biomedical Informatics
University of Utah

Vicente Planelles, Ph.D.
Professor
Division of Microbiology and Immunology
Department of Pathology
University of Utah School of Medicine
Salt Lake City, UT

Travis Norseth
MD Candidate Class of 2021
University of Utah School of Medicine
Salt Lake City, UT

Naveen Rathi
MD Candidate Class of 2021
University of Utah School of Medicine
Salt Lake City, UT

David Ortiz
MD Candidate Class of 2021
University of Utah School of Medicine
Salt Lake City, UT

REPRODUCTIVE EMBRYOLOGY

Section I - Early Fetal Development

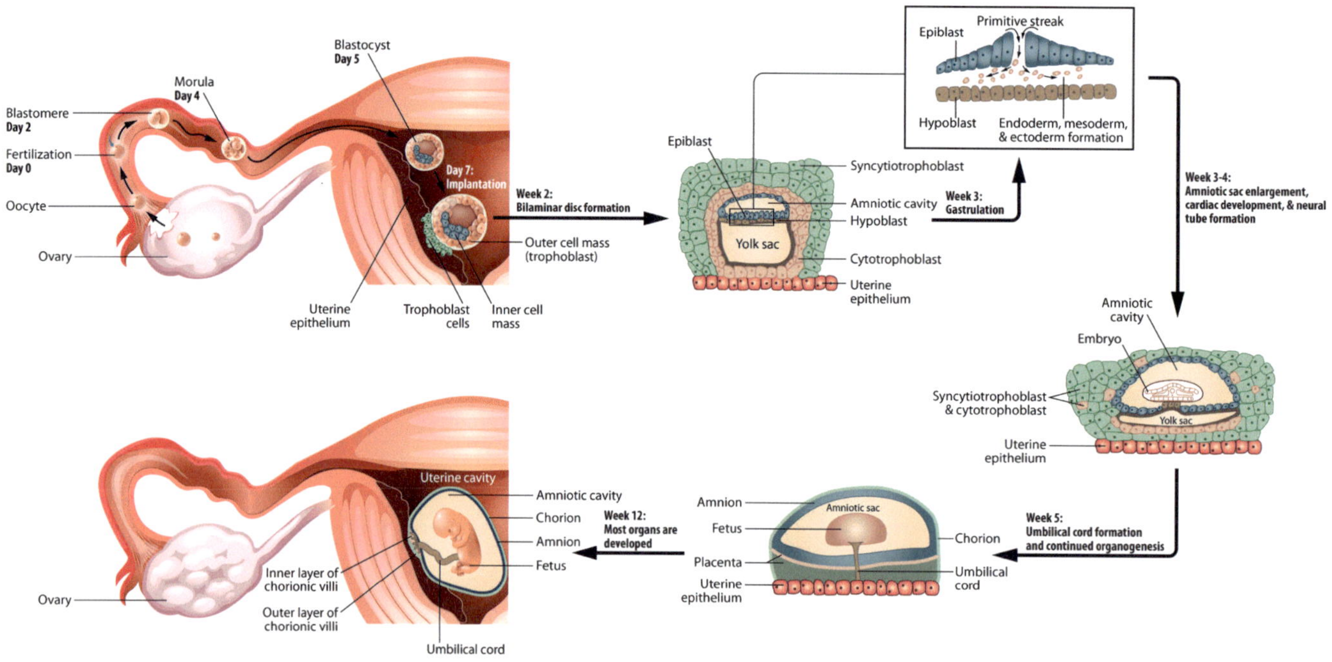

Figure 6.1.1 - Early fetal development overview

I. Week 2
   A. Week 2 = 2 layers
   B. Bilaminar disc
      1. Epiblast
      2. Hypoblast

II. Week 3
   A. Week 3 = 3 layers
   B. Epiblast invaginates → primitive streak
   C. Gastrulation occurs → endoderm, mesoderm, and ectoderm

III. Weeks 3 - 4
   A. Amniotic sac enlargement
   B. Cardiac development
   C. Neural tube formation
   D. Limb buds form
   E. Very susceptible to teratogens (weeks 3-8)

IV. Weeks 5 - 12
   A. Week 6
      1. Fetal cardiac activity visible via transvaginal ultrasound

B. Week 8

1. Fetal movements begins

C. Week 10

1. Genitalia have male or female characteristics

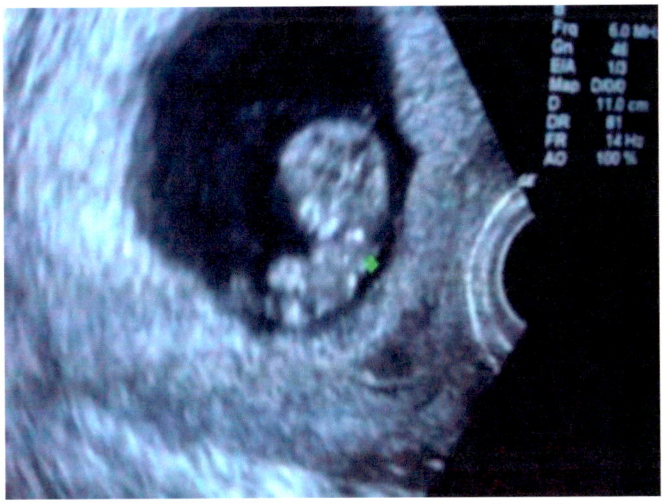

Figure 6.1.2 - Normal ultrasound of a 10-week-old fetus

REVIEW QUESTIONS

1. A 24-year-old pregnant woman comes to the clinic due to dysuria and urgency that began yesterday. She states that she has leftover pills of TMP-SMX (Bactrim) from a previous UTI infection and is wondering if she can take this medication. If she takes this medication, at what stage in development would her baby be most susceptible to the adverse effects of Bactrim?

   A. 1-4 days
   B. 6-10 days
   C. 2 weeks
   D. 4-6 weeks
   E. 10-12 weeks

- **Correct answer: D**
- **TMP-SMX has teratogenic effects.**
- **Fetuses are most susceptible to teratogens during the embryonic period of 3-8 weeks because this is when important organs are forming.**
- **A is incorrect. 1-4 days is when the egg is fertilized and divides to become the morula.**
- **B is incorrect. 6 -10 days is when the blastocyst implants and begins secreting hCG.**
- **C is incorrect. At two weeks the bilaminar disc has formed.**
- **E is incorrect. After 8 weeks a lot of the basic organogenesis has occurred so the embryo is not as susceptible to teratogens.**

Section II - Genes of Body Patterning

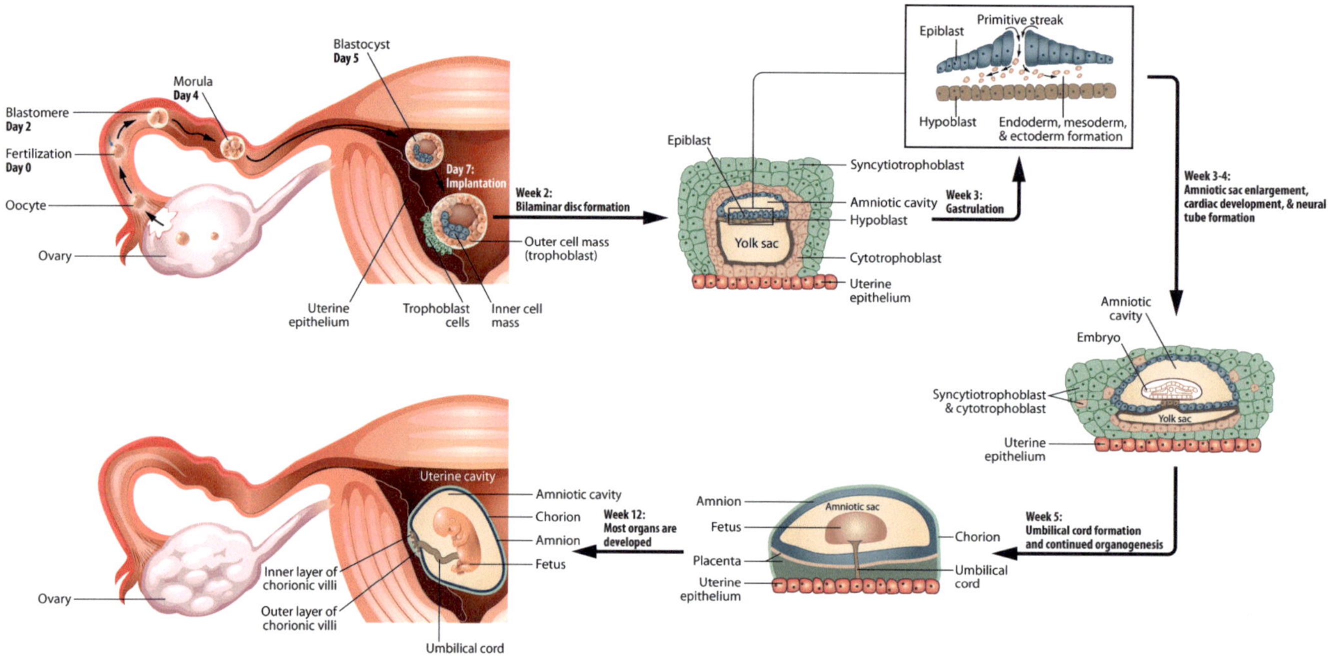

Figure 6.1.1 - Early fetal development overview

Genes	Function	Notes
Fibroblast growth factor (FGF)	• Proximal-distal limb development (limb elongation)	• Produced by apical ectodermal ridge (AER)
Wnt-7	• Dorsal-ventral limb development • Wnt-7 → dorsal development • Lack of Wnt-7 → ventral development	• Produced by apical ectodermal ridge (AER)
Homeobox (Hox)	• Produce transcription factors • Organizes body segments in craniocaudal direction • Anterior-posterior limb development (eg, “place an arm here with 5 fingers”)	• Mutations can lead to body parts in abnormal locations, polydactyly, or syndactyly
Sonic hedgehog (SHH)	• Anterior-posterior limb development (eg, “make this 5th digit short”) • Separates forebrain into right and left hemispheres	• Mutations can lead to holoprosencephaly

Table 6.1.1 - Genes of body patterning

Limb Orientation

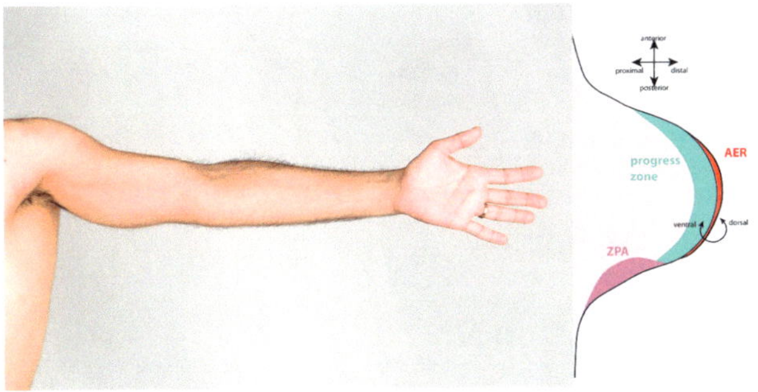

Genusfotografen (genusfotografen.se) &; Wikimedia Sverige (wikimedia.se) [CC BY-SA 4.0] Terrasigillata at English Wikipendia [CC BY-SA 3.0]

Figure 6.1.3 - Limb orientation

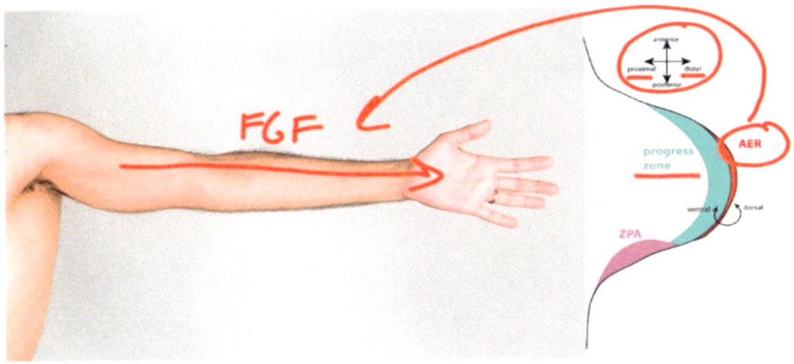

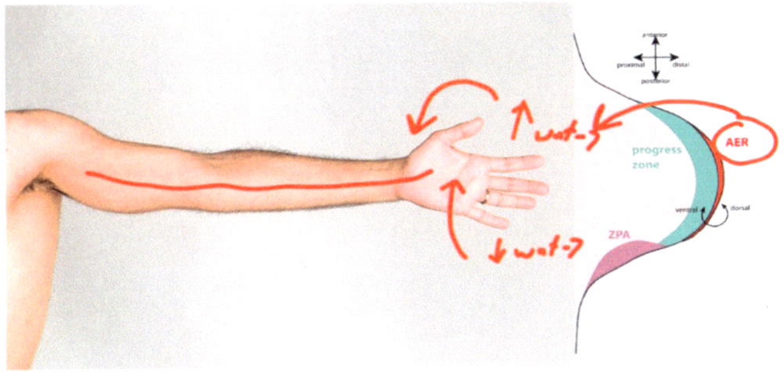

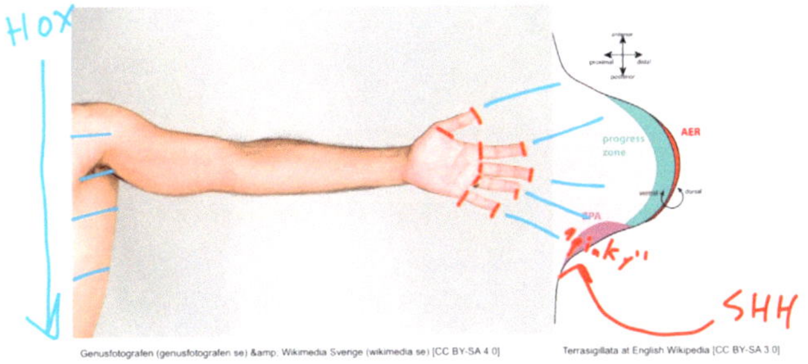

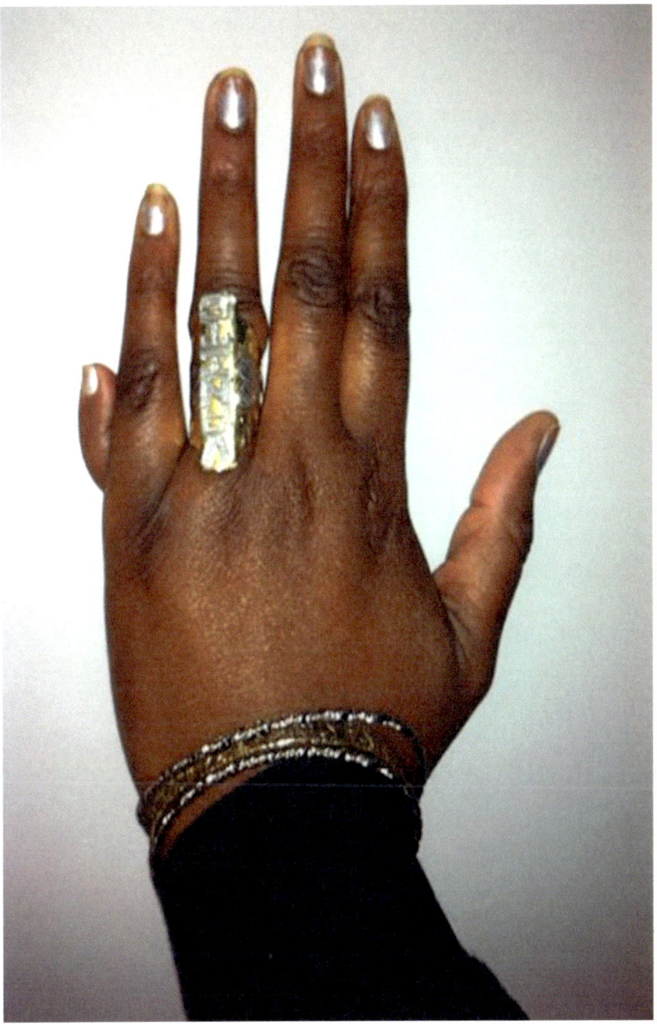

Photo credit: Cplbeaudoin at English Wikipedia [CC BY-SA 3.0 (https://creativecommons.org/licenses/by-sa/3.0)]

Figure 6.1.4 - Polydactyly

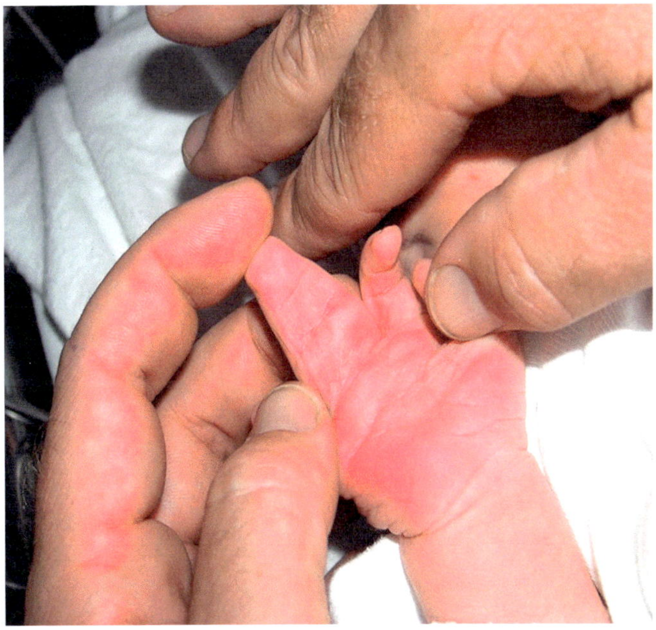

Photo Credit: Dumplestilskin, uploaded by Gliu [Public domain]

Figure 6.1.5 - Syndactyly

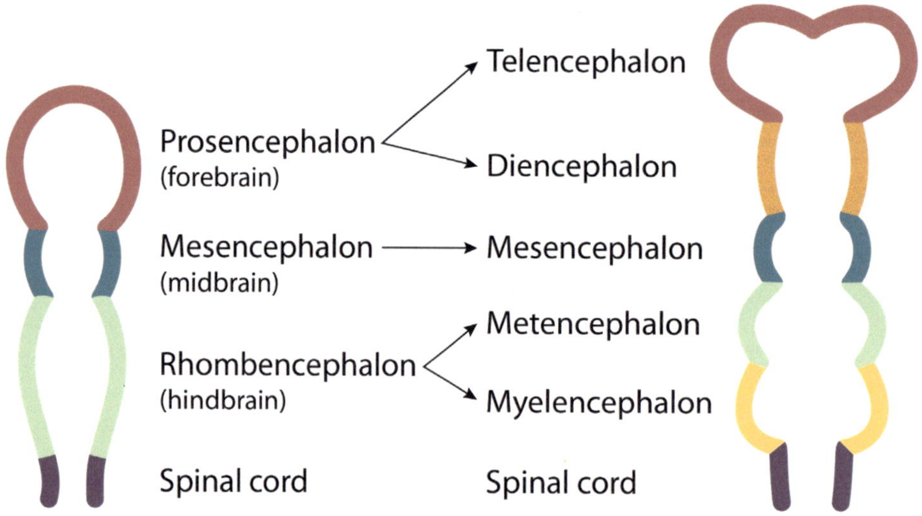

Figure 6.1.6 - Brain segments and cavities derived from the neural tube

I. Holoprosencephaly

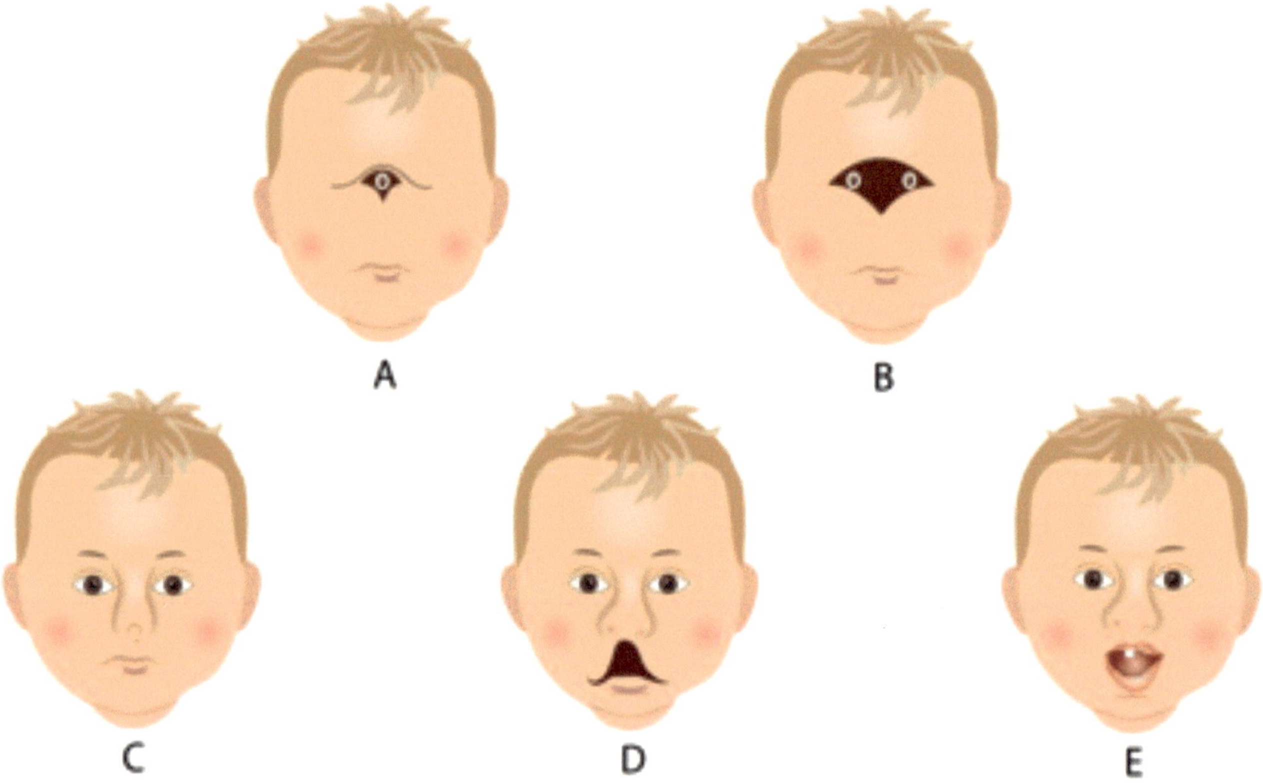

Figure 6.1.7 - Spectrum of midline defects and holoprosencephaly

REVIEW QUESTIONS

1. A baby is born with forearm flexor muscles where extensor muscles should have been. This abnormality was most likely caused by under secretion of a molecule normally secreted from which of the following?

   A. Zone of polarizing action
   B. Apical ectodermal ridge
   C. Progress zone
   D. Mesoderm
   E. Endoderm

- **Answer: B, apical ectodermal ridge**
- **Flexor muscles on the dorsal surface of the forearm indicates abnormal ventralization.**
- **Dorsal-ventral patterning is determined by Wnt-7 which is produced from the apical ectodermal ridge**
- **A and C are incorrect because these zones do not produce the Wnt-7 protein**
- **D and E are incorrect because the apical ectodermal ridge is ectoderm**

Section III - Embryologic Derivatives

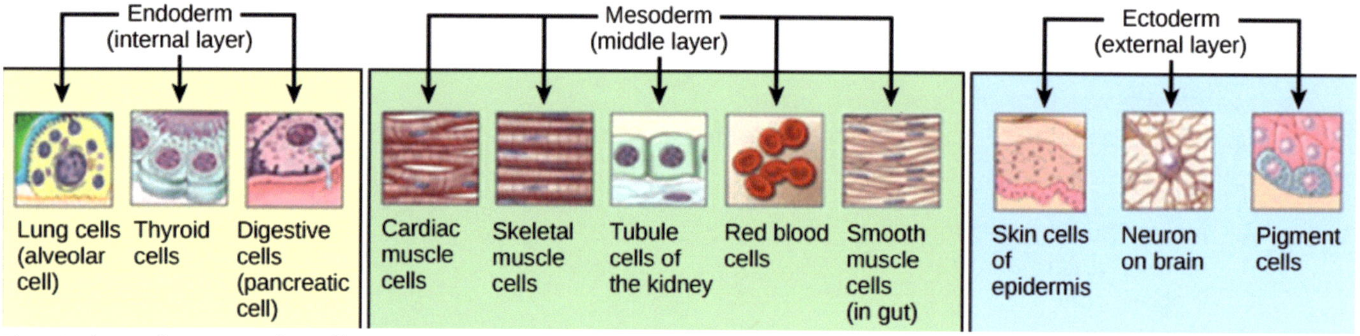

Photo Credit: CNX [CC BY-SA 3.0 (https://creativecommons.org/licenses/by-sa/3.0)]

Figure 6.1.8 - Embryological derivatives

I. Endoderm
   A. "Enternal" layer
      1. Gut tube epithelium
      2. Liver, gallbladder, pancreas
      3. Most of urethra and lower vagina
      4. Lungs
      5. Cells of thyroid and parathyroid
      6. Eustachian tubes
      7. Thymus

II. Mesoderm
   A. Mesoderm = middle layer
      1. Muscle, bone, connective tissue
      2. Serous lining of cavities
      3. Spleen
      4. Cardiovascular
      5. Blood and lymphatics
      6. Wall of gut tube
      7. Upper vagina, testes, ovaries
      8. Kidneys, adrenal cortex

III. Mesodermal Defects
   A. "VACTERL" associations
      1. Vertebral anomalies
      2. Anal atresia
      3. Cardiac defect
      4. TE fistula
      5. Renal defects
      6. Limb defects
   B. Association = group of birth defects that co-occur with no pathologic explanation

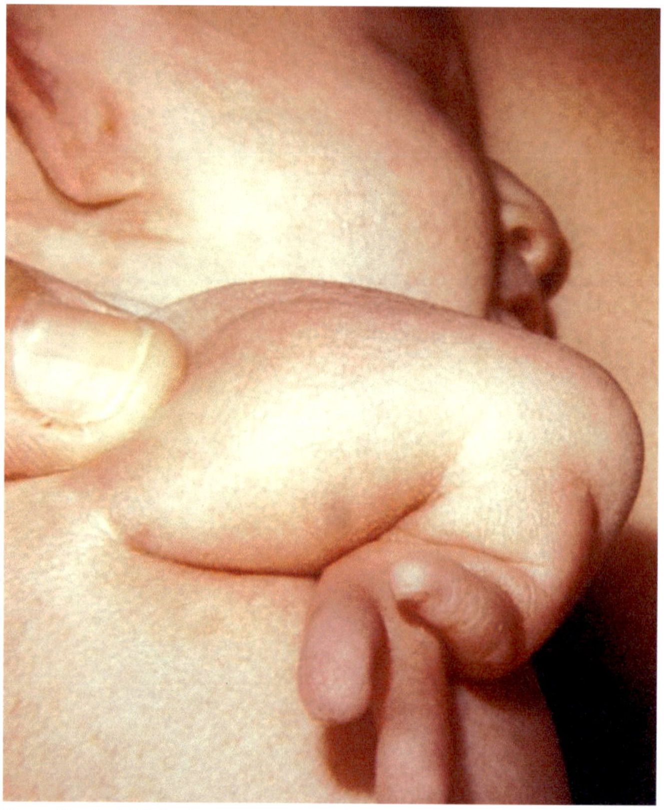

Photo Credit: CDC/Dr. James W. Hanson [Public domain]

Figure 6.1.9 - Mesodermal defect

IV. Surface Ectoderm

A. External layer

1. Epidermis
2. Anterior pituitary (Rathke pouch)
3. Sensory organs
4. Lens of eye
5. Epithelial lining of oral cavity
6. Anal canal below pectinate line
7. Glands: parotid, sweat, mammary

V. Neural Tube

A. Central nervous system

1. Brain
2. Retina
3. Spinal cord

B. Part of the neuroectoderm

C. Failure of the neural tube to fuse → neural tube defects

D. Folic acid is important

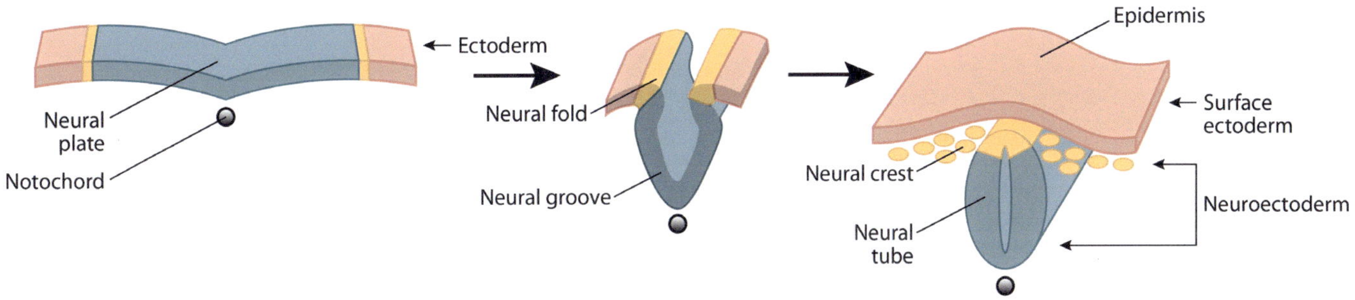

Figure 6.1.10 - Neurulation

VI. Neural Crest

A. Mnemonic: "MOTEL PASSES"

B. Melanocytes

C. Odontoblasts

D. Tracheal lining

E. Enterochromaffin cells

F. Leptomeninges

G. PNS ganglia

H. Adrenal medulla

I. Schwann cells

J. Spiral membrane

K. Endocardial cushions

L. Skull bones

REVIEW QUESTIONS

?

1. A 7-year-old boy is brought to the physician due to shortness of breath and chest pain. Upon further investigation he is given a diagnosis of sickle cell disease. What is the embryologic derivative of the cells affected by individuals with this condition?

    - **The correct answer is mesoderm.**
    - **This boy has sickle cell disease. In this disorder the red blood cells are affected and red blood cells are derived from mesoderm.**

Section IV - Errors in Morphogenesis

I. Morphogenesis

A. Morphogenesis: the biological process that causes an organism to develop its shape

II. Type of Errors

A. Intrinsic

1. Failure of embryo to develop due to abnormal genes or other internal processes
2. Agenesis, aplasia, hypoplasia, malformation

B. Extrinsic

1. External factors within the womb disrupt normal development
2. Deformation, disruption

III. Agenesis

A. Absent organ due to absent primordial tissue

B. Renal agenesis → oligohydramnios → Potter sequence

1. Pulmonary hypoplasia
2. Flat facies
3. Clubfeet
4. Wrinkly skin

IV. Aplasia

A. An absent organ despite the presence of primordial tissue

B. DiGeorge syndrome = thymic aplasia

1. Failure to develop 3rd and 4th pharyngeal pouches
2. Thymic, parathyroid, & cardiac defects

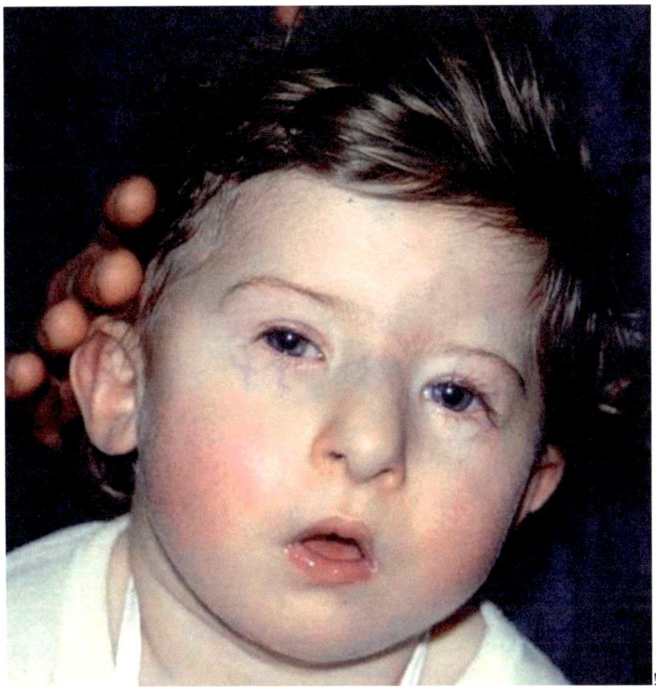

Figure 6.1.11 - Abnormal facies of a patient with DiGeorge syndrome

V. Hypoplasia

A. Underdevelopment or incomplete development of an organ or tissue

B. Klinefelter syndrome

1. 47, XXY
2. Testicular hypoplasia
3. Results in low testosterone

VI. Malformation

A. Occurs when a structure is not formed, partially formed, or abnormally formed during embryonic development (weeks 3-8)

B. Holoprosencephaly

1. Forebrain development
2. Midline defects
3. CNS deformities

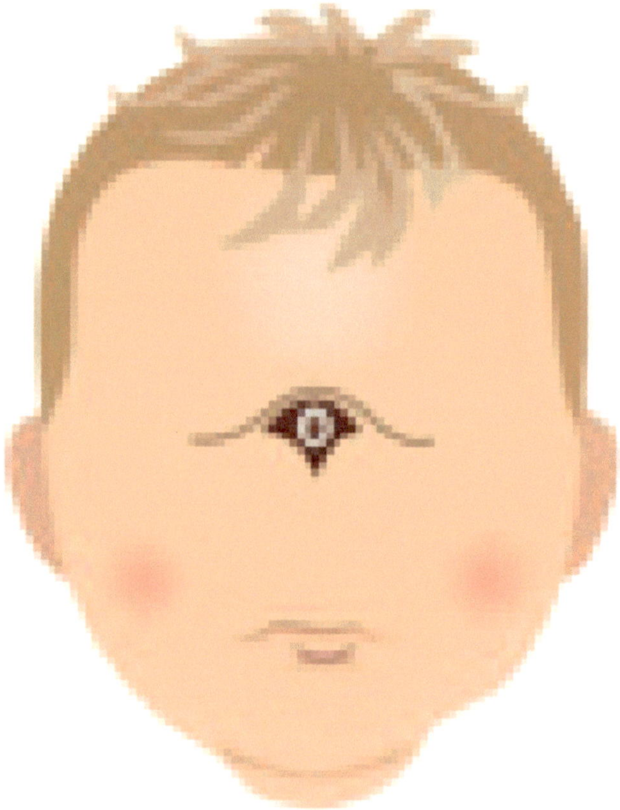

Figure 6.1.12 - Cyclopia

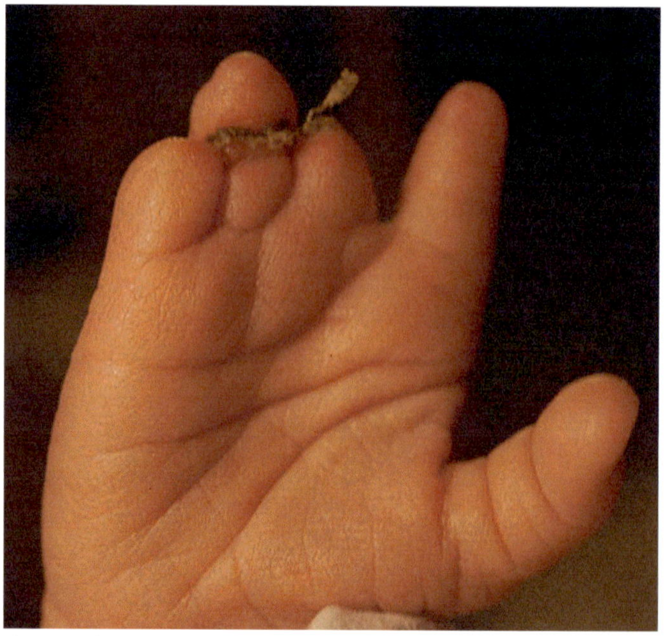

Photo Credit: Moscowmom [Public domain]

Figure 6.1.13 - Amniotic band sequence

VII. Deformation

A. Abnormality of the position of body parts due to extrinsic intrauterine mechanical forces

B. Occurs after embryonic period (weeks 3-8)

C. Septate or bicornuate uterus

1. Fetal compression
2. Flattened skull

VIII. Disruption

A. Secondary breakdown of previously normal tissue or structure

B. Can result from vascular or mechanical process that leads to tissue compromise

C. Amniotic band sequence (ABS)

1. Constrictive rings
2. Limb defects

REVIEW QUESTIONS

1. A 3-day-old boy is brought to the clinic by his mother due to difficulty feeding. She is worried that he is starving and nothing she does helps him feed better. On physical examination, the newborn is well-appearing but is found to have a cleft palate. What type of error of morphogenesis best describes this patient's presentation?

   A. Agenesis
   B. Aplasia
   C. Hypoplasia
   D. Malformation
   E. Deformation

- **The correct answer is D.**
- **A cleft palate occurs when a structure is partially or abnormally formed and is a midline defect.**
- **This falls into the category of a malformation, so D is the correct answer**
- **A and B are incorrect. Agenesis and aplasia are incorrect because there is no organ missing.**
- **C is incorrect. Hypoplasia is incorrect because again, all organs appear to have developed normally and there is no mention of underdevelopment, but rather abnormal development.**
- **E is incorrect. Deformation is incorrect because deformations are due to extrinsic forces, while a cleft palate is an intrinsic error.**

Section V - Teratogens

I. Teratogens

  A. Teratogen = an agent that causes abnormalities of the developing fetus

  B. Fetus is most susceptible during weeks 3-8 of pregnancy

  C. Mechanisms:

    1. Induce cell death

    2. Alter normal growth of tissues

    3. Interfere with cellular differentiation

  D. Severity depends on amount, duration, and genetics

Teratogen	Pathophysiology	Clinical Outcome
Diethylstilbestrol (DES)	• Disrupts Müllerian duct epithelium in utero	• Vaginal clear cell adenocarcinoma • Various reproductive tract abnormalities and infertility
Thalidomide	• Blocks vascular angiogenesis in fetal limbs	• Stunted or malformed limbs
Radiation (high dose)	• Ionizing radiation disrupts growth of neural tissue and other tissues (diagnostic radiation is not considered high dose radiation)	• Intellectual disability and microcephaly
Methylmercury (organic mercury)	• High doses come from many types of fish and are toxic to the developing brain	• Cerebral palsy and developmental delay

Table 6.1.2 - Teratogens

Drug
ACE inhibitors
Alkylating agents (cyclophosphamide, busulfan, ifosfamide, nitrosoureas)
Aminoglycosides
Phenytoin
Carbamazepine
Valproate
Methotrexate
Isotretinoin (Accutane) or excess vitamin A
Lithium
Methimazole
Iodine deficiency
Tetracyclines
Warfarin
Alcohol
Nicotine
Cocaine
Opioids
Marijuana
Maternal diabetes

Table 6.1.3 - Other teratogens covered in pharmacology

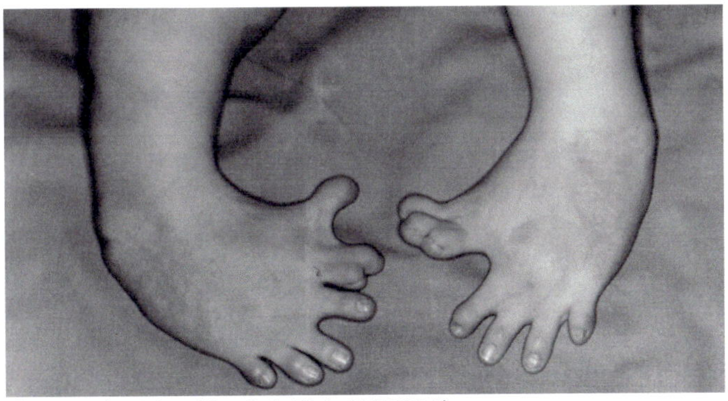

Photo Credit: Otisarchives3 via Flickr (CC BY 2.0)

Figure 6.1.14 - Foot malformations with thalidomide

REVIEW QUESTIONS

1. A 2-year-old girl is unable to walk because she cannot lift her lower left limb. The girl's mother states the patient has never moved her left leg, even as an infant when getting her diaper changed. Both upper and lower limbs are otherwise normal-appearing. Which teratogenic exposure is more likely to cause this presentation: thalidomide or organic mercury?

    - **Answer: Organic mercury**
    - **Organic mercury, or methylmercury, is known to damage the developing motor cortex, leading to cerebral palsy, which is seen in this patient**
    - **Thalidomide can cause malformed limbs, but not paralysis as seen in this patient**

Section VI - Twinning

I. Dizygotic vs. Monozygotic

A. Dizygotic (fraternal)

1. Two separate eggs, each fertilized with its own sperm
2. More common than monozygotic twins
3. Common in IVF

B. Monozygotic (identical)

1. One fertilized egg that splits in early pregnancy

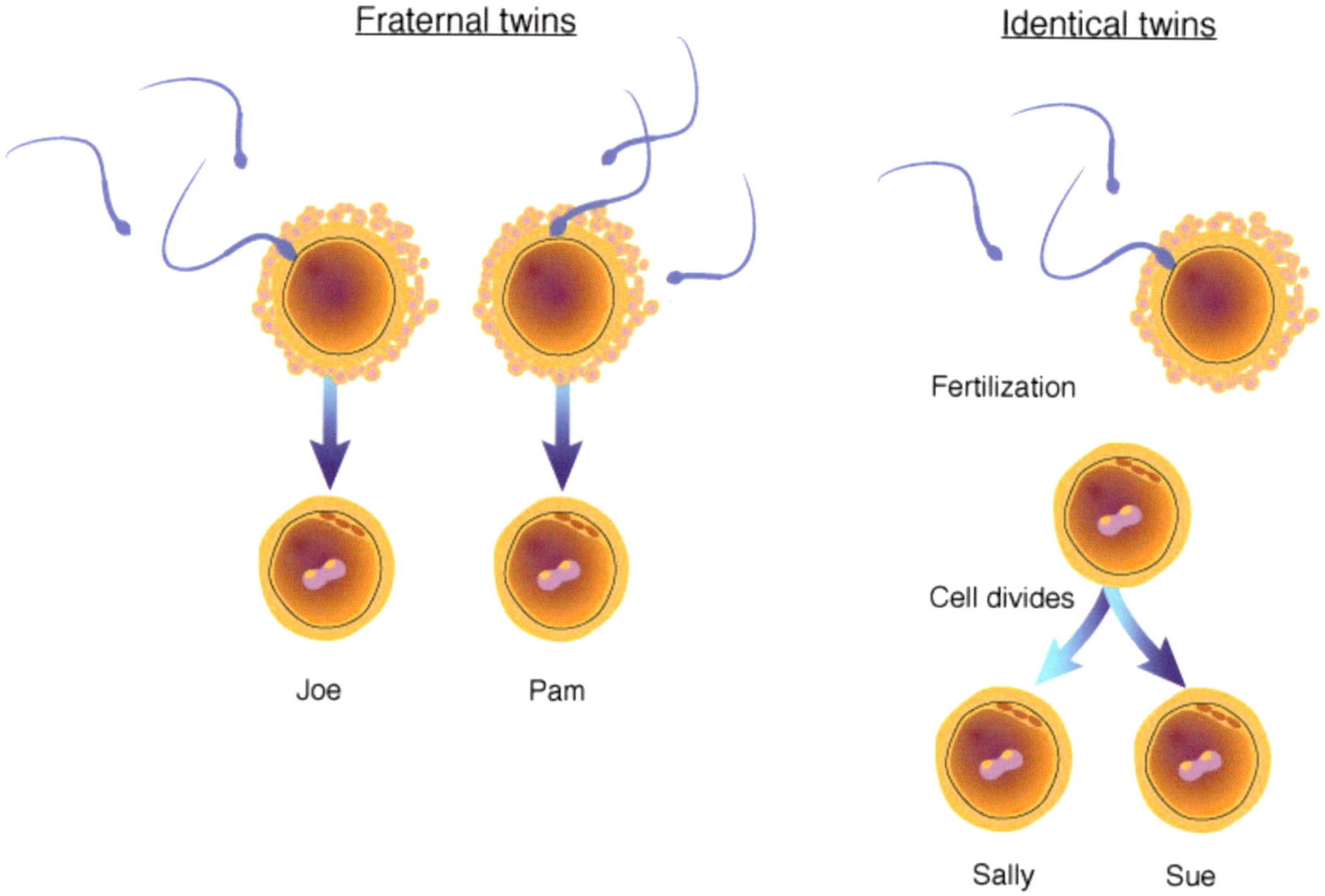

Photo Credit: Public Domain

Figure 6.1.15 - Chorionicity and amnionicity during fetal development

II. Chorionicity and Amnionicity of Dizygotic Twins

A. Zygotes form and develop separately → dichorionic, diamniotic

III. Chorionicity and Amnionicity of Monozygotic Twins

A. S (separate): division during 2-cell to morula stage (< 5 days) → dichorionic, diamniotic

B. C (chorion shared): division of blastocyst (days 5-8) → monochorionic, diamniotic

C. This is the most common at 75% ("C" for "common")

D. A (amnion shared): division of bilaminar disc (days 8-12) → monochorionic, monoamniotic

E. B (body shared, conjoined): division of trilaminar disc (days 13+) → monochorionic, monoamniotic, and conjoined

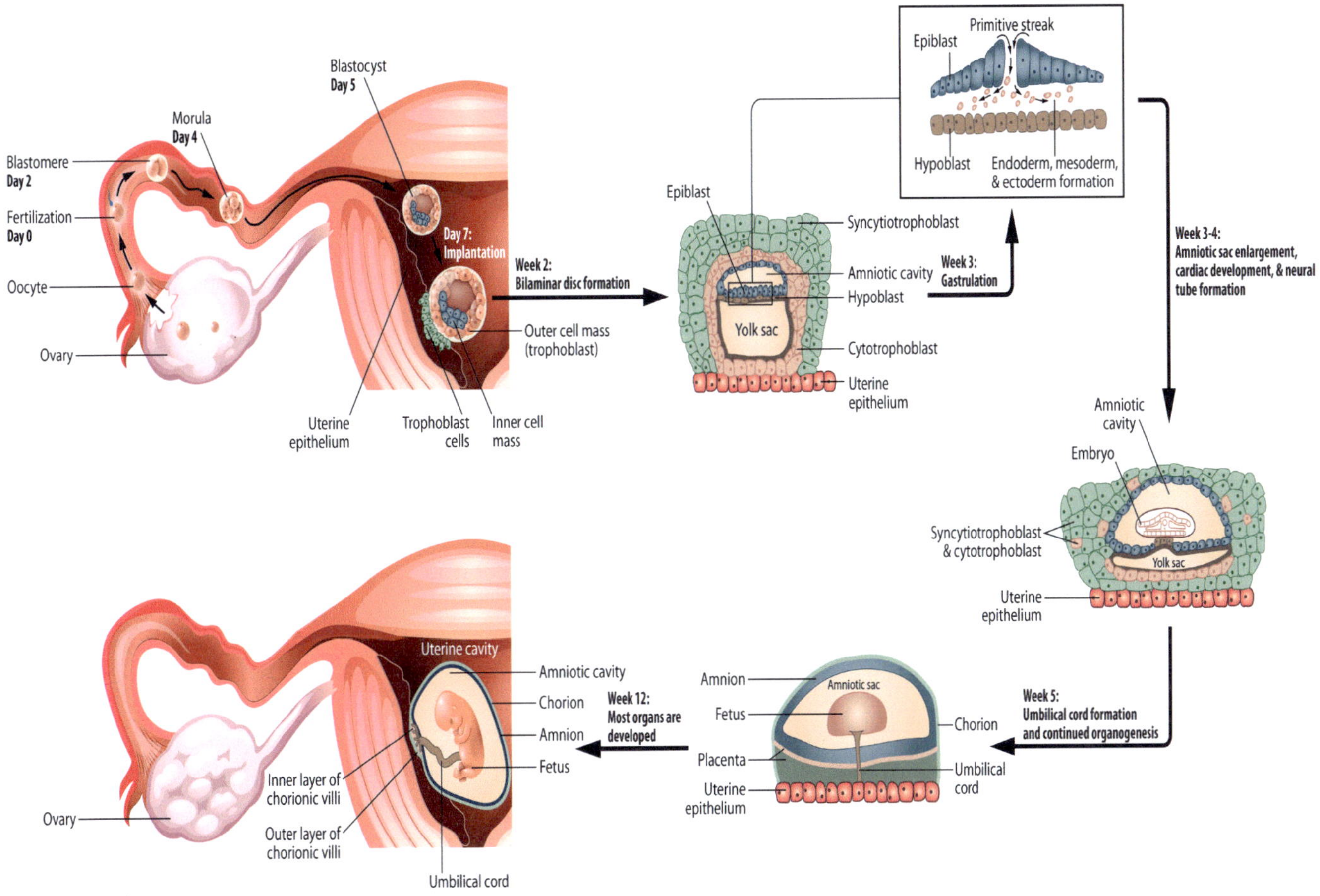

Figure 6.1.1 - Early fetal development overview

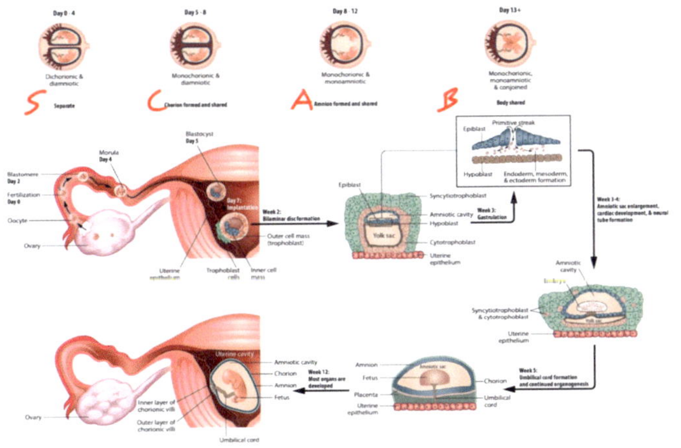

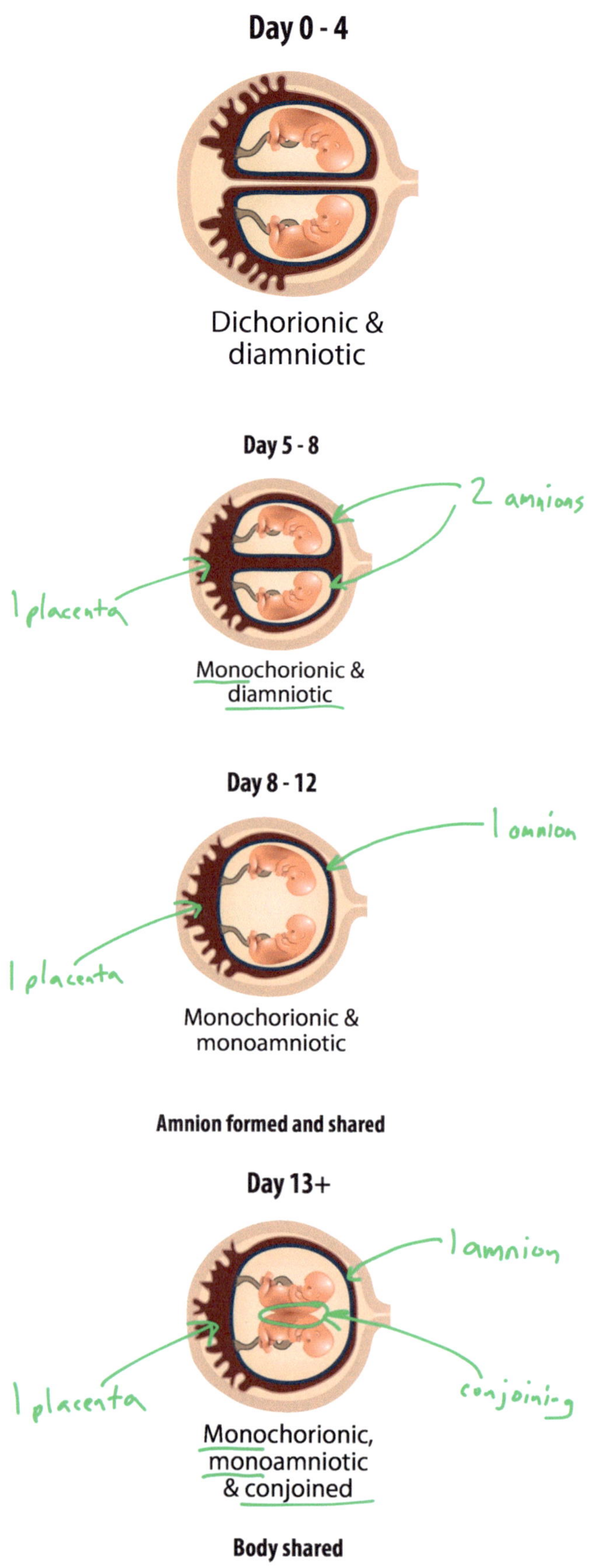

Figure 1.16

REVIEW QUESTIONS ?

1. A developing embryo splits on day 10 of gestation. What structure(s) will most likely be shared by the developing twins?

- **Answer: The amnion and chorion (placenta**
- **Remember the mnemonic SCAB**
  - **Separate - splitting before day 5**
  - **Chorion (placenta) - splitting between days 5-8**
  - **Amnion - splitting between days 8-12**
  - **And body - splitting on day 13 or after**
    - **Splitting on day 10 (falls between days 8-12) indicates that the twins will share the amnion as well as the chorion which has already developed**
    - **So these twins will be monochorionic and monoamniotic**

Section VII - Pharyngeal Clefts and Pouches

I. Pharyngeal Apparatus

A. Mnemonic: CAP

1. Clefts (grooves) = ectoderm
2. Arches = mesoderm and neural crest cells
3. Pouches = endoderm

II. Pharyngeal Clefts

A. 1st cleft

1. External auditory meatus

B. 2nd - 4th clefts

1. Temporary cervical sinuses → obliterated

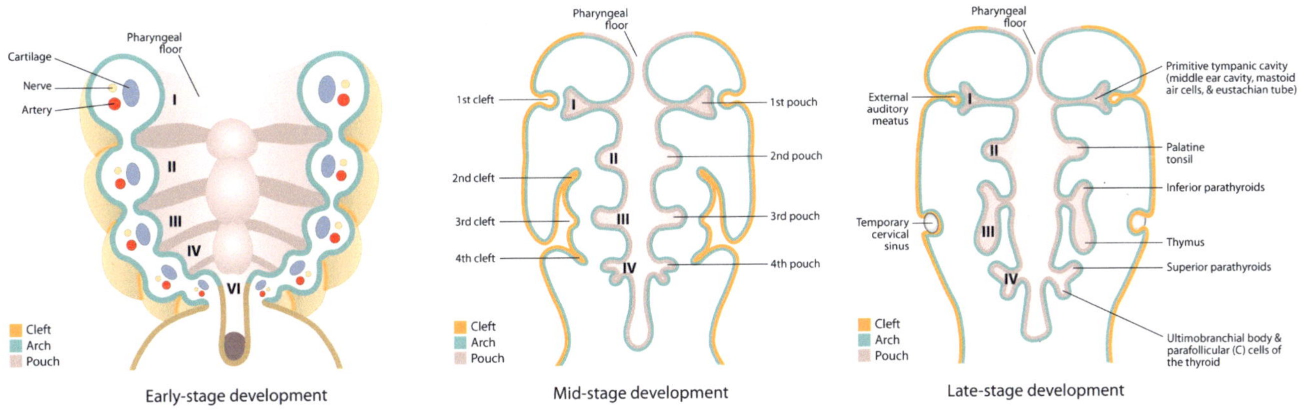

Figure 6.1.17 - Pharyngeal apparatus development

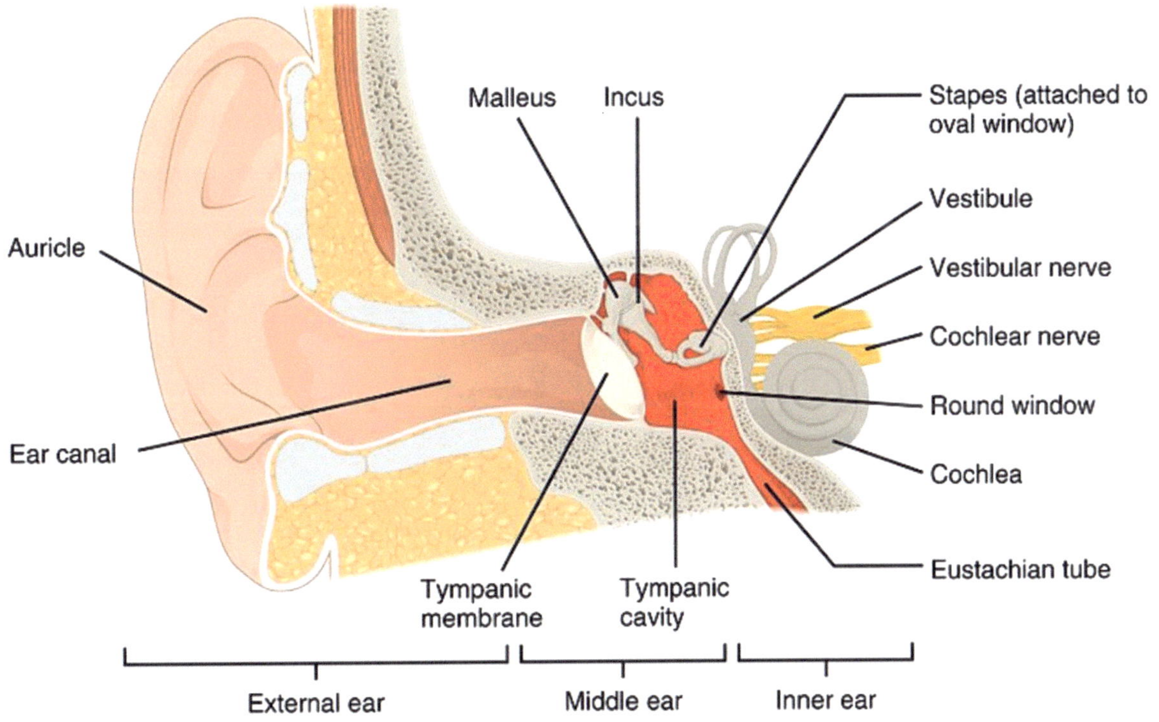

Figure 6.1.18 - Adult human ear

III. Branchial Cleft Cyst

A. Failure of the temporary cervical sinus to obliterate

B. More common in children (rare in adults)

C. Neck mass located anterior to the sternocleidomastoid muscle (lateral neck region)

D. Often confused with cancer

E. Mass is immovable when swallowing

F. Must differentiate from a thyroglossal duct cyst (midline immovable mass)

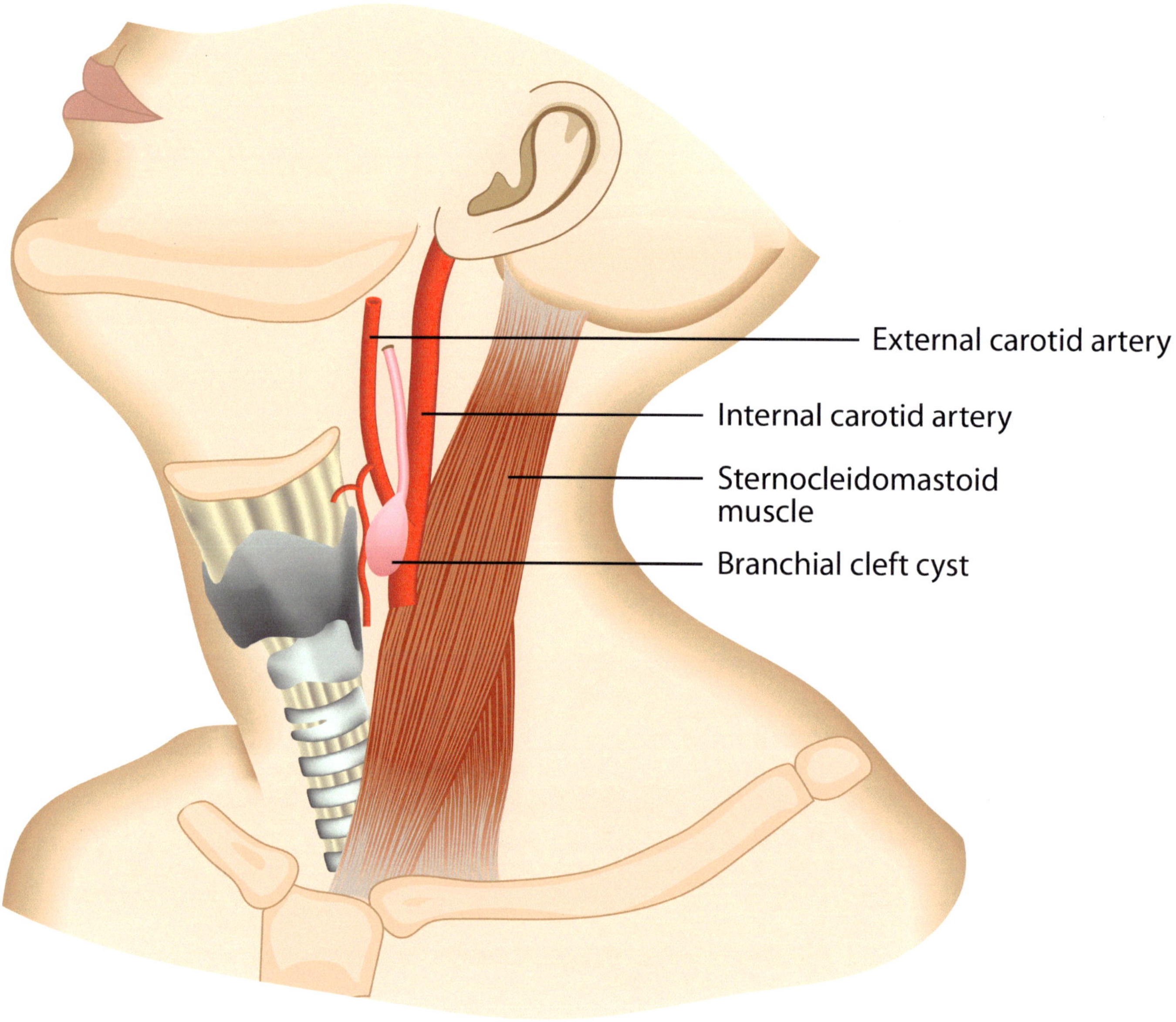

Figure 6.1.19 - Branchial cleft cyst

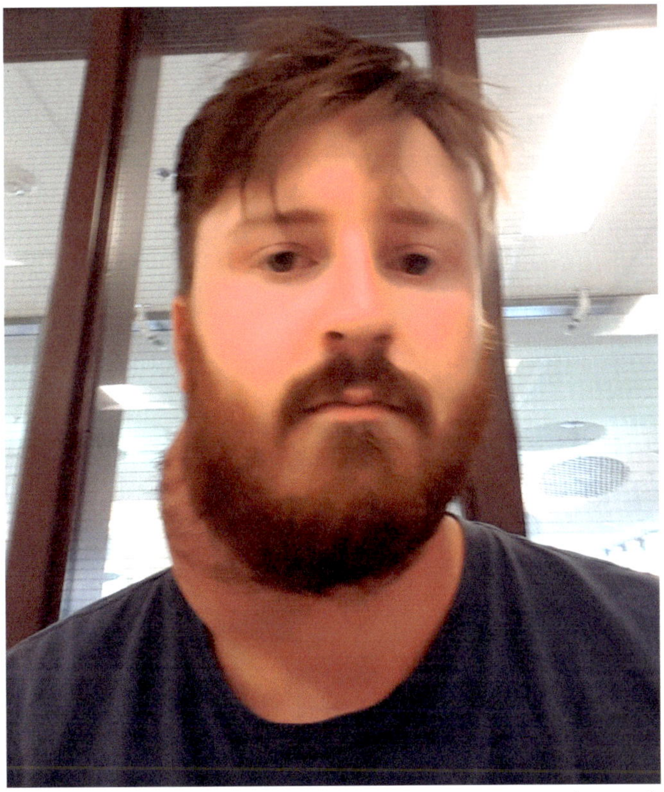

Figure 6.1.20 - Patient with a branchial cleft cyst

Pharyngeal Pouch	Derivatives
1st	• Middle ear cavity, eustachian tube, and mastoid air cells
2nd	• Palatine tonsil
3rd	• Dorsal wings: inferior parathyroids • Ventral wings: thymus
4th	• Dorsal wings: superior parathyroids • Ventral wings: ultimopharyngeal body → parafollicular C cells of the thyroid

Table 6.1.4 - Pharyngeal pouch derivatives

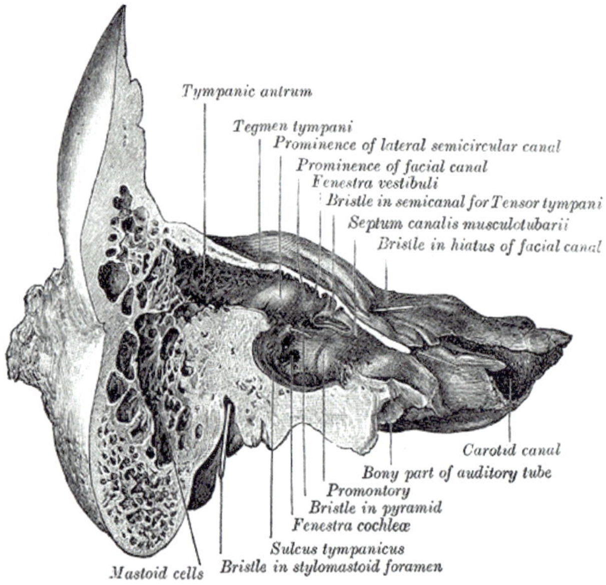

Photo Credit: Henry Vandyke Carter [Public domain]

Figure 6.1.21 - Coronal section of the temporal bone and ear

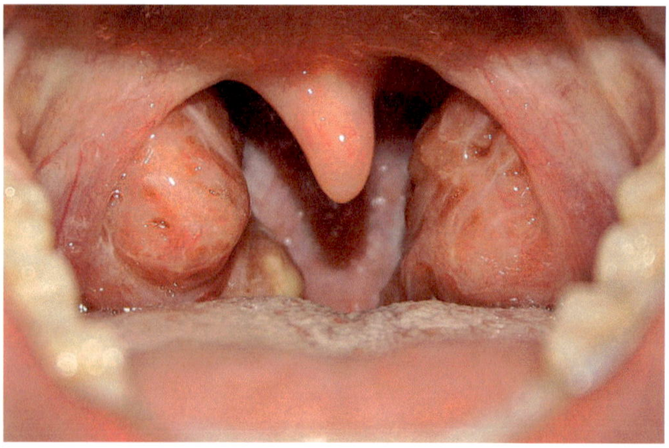

Photo Credit: Klem [CC BY 3.0 (https://creativecommons.org/licenses/by/3.0)]

Figure 6.1.22 - Palatine tonsils

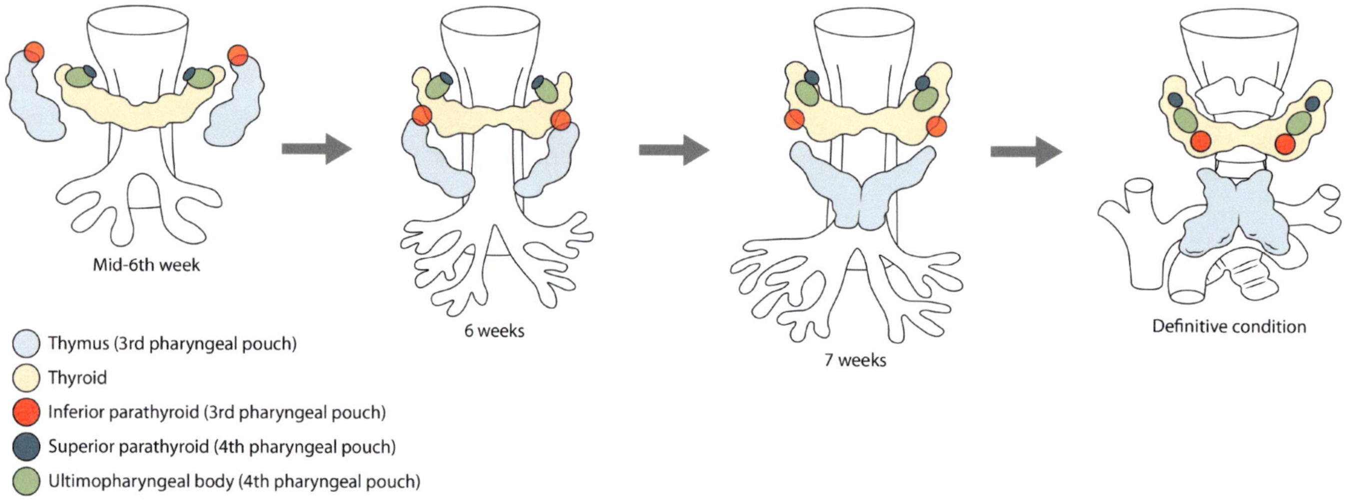

Figure 6.1.23 - Movement of the 3rd and 4th pharyngeal pouches

REVIEW QUESTIONS

1. A 3-year-old boy is brought to clinic because he has been displaying muscle weakness, fatigue, tingling in his fingers, and frequent infections. A complete metabolic panel reveals a low calcium level. Blood work also shows a T-cell deficiency. If these conditions are caused by a defect in the pharyngeal apparatus, malformation of which of the following structures would most likely cause his symptoms?

   A. 1st and 2nd arch
   B. 3rd and 4th arch
   C. 4th and 6th arch
   D. 1st and 2nd pouch
   E. 3rd and 4th pouch

- **The correct answer is E.**
- **The 2 main issues are hypocalcemia and t-cell deficiency.**
- **The pharyngeal pouches give rise to the parathyroid glands and thymus. A problem in these two would definitely lead to the symptoms seen in the boy, because the parathyroid gland helps regulate calcium levels and the thymus aids in T-cell development.**
- **Specifically the thymus and parathyroid glands are derived from the 3rd and 4th pouch so in this case the correct answer is E.**
- **A is incorrect. The 1st and 2nd arches give rise to a lot of structures in the face, including the maxillary artery, the muscles of mastication, the muscles of facial expression, and branches of the facial and trigeminal nerve. However, defects in any of these would not lead to hypocalcemia or a T-cell deficiency.**
- **B is incorrect. The 3rd and 4th arches give rise to the stylopharyngeus, pharyngeal and laryngeal musculature, branches of the vagus nerve and glossopharyngeal. Defects in any of these would not lead to hypocalcemia or T-cell deficiency.**
- **C is incorrect. The 4th and 6th arch gives rise to arytenoid cartilages, laryngeal musculature and branches of the vagus nerve. These would not cause the child's symptoms. The 1st pouch gives rise to the Middle ear cavity, eustachian tube, and mastoid air cells and the 2nd pouch to the palatine tonsils. None of these would cause his symptoms. Only the 3rd and 4th pouch would as these give rise to the thymus and parathyroid glands.**

Section VIII - 1st and 2nd Pharyngeal Arches

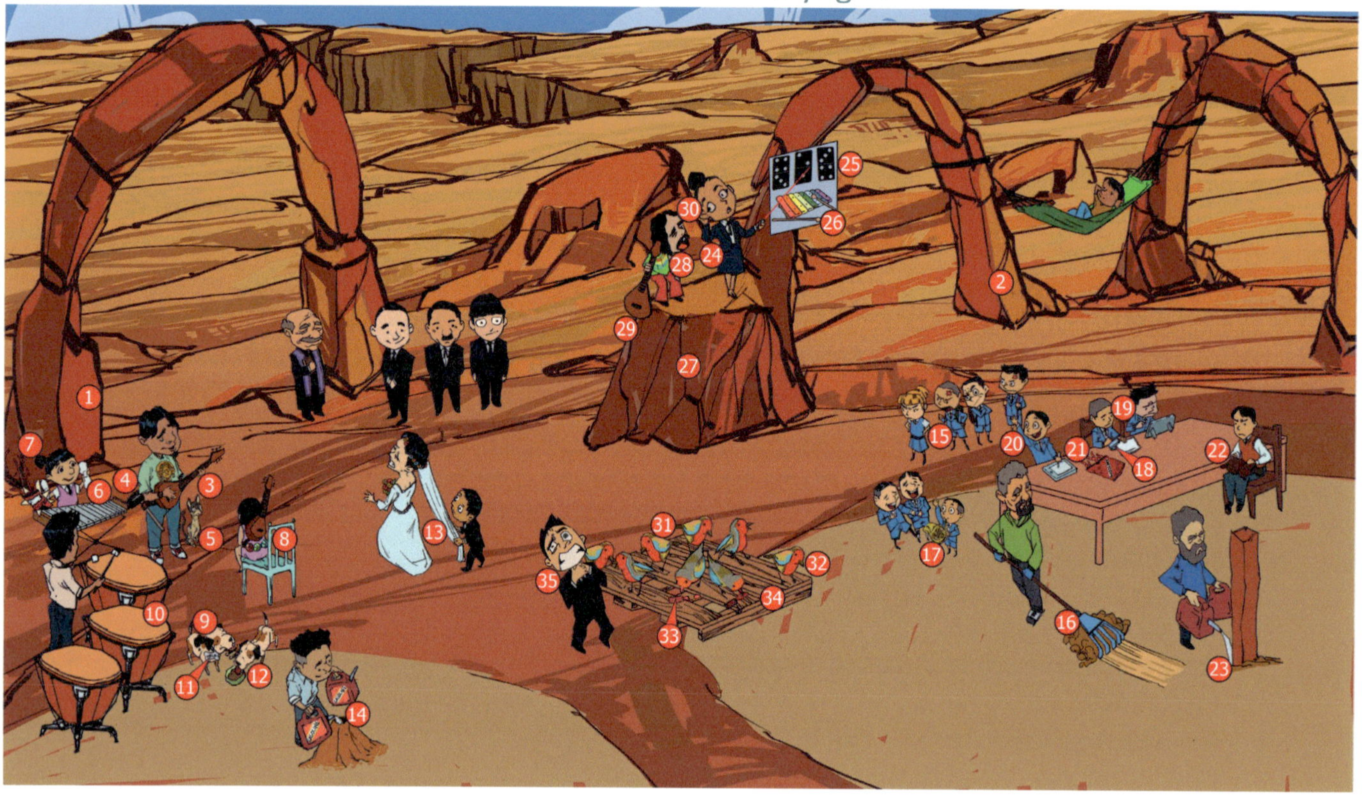

1. ______________________________
2. ______________________________
3. ______________________________
4. ______________________________
5. ______________________________
6. ______________________________
7. ______________________________
8. ______________________________
9. ______________________________
10. ______________________________
11. ______________________________
12. ______________________________
13. ______________________________
14. ______________________________
15. ______________________________
16. ______________________________
17. ______________________________
18. ______________________________

Arch	Cartilage	Muscles	Nerves	Arteries
1st	- **Maxillary process**: maxilla, zygomatic bone - **Mandibular process**: mandible, Meckel's cartilage (malleus, incus), and sphenomandibular ligament	- **Muscles of mastication** (temporalis, masseter, and lateral and medial pterygoids) - Mylohyoid, anterior belly of digastric, tensor tympani, anterior ⅔ of tongue, and tensor veli palatini	- CN V_3	- Maxillary artery
2nd	- **Reichert's cartilage**: stapes, styloid, lesser horn of hyoid, stylohyoid ligament	- **Muscles of facial expression**: stapedius, stylohyoid, platysma, posterior belly of digastric	- CN VII	- Stapedial artery - Hyoid artery
3rd	- Greater horn of hyoid	- Stylopharyngeus - Posterior ⅓ of tongue	- CN IX	- Common carotid arteries - Proximal part of internal carotid
4th	- Arytenoids, cricoid, corniculate, cuneiform, and thyroid	- Cricothyroid, levator veli palatini, pharyngeal constrictors, and the posterior ⅓ of the tongue	- CN X (superior laryngeal branch)	- Left: aortic arch - Right: proximal part of subclavian artery
6th		- Intrinsic muscles of larynx (except cricothyroid)	- CN X (inferior laryngeal branch)	- Proximal part of pulmonary arteries - Ductus arteriosus

Table 6.1.5 - Pharyngeal arches

I. Disorders

   A. Treacher Collins syndrome

   B. Pierre Robin sequence

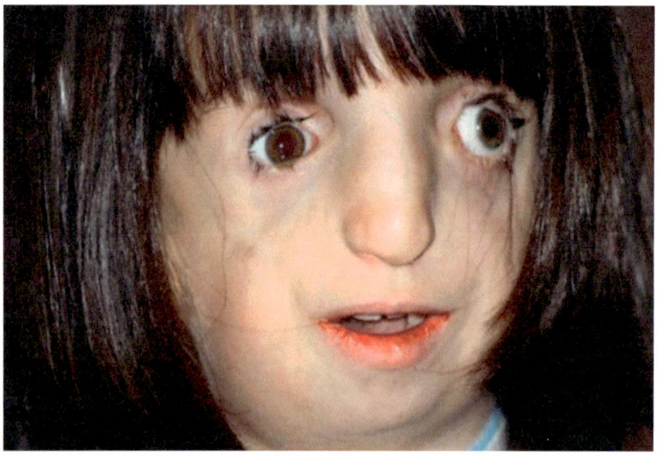

Photo Credit: Article of MedMedicine [CC BY-SA 4.0 (https://creativecommons.org/licenses/by-sa/4.0)]

Figure 6.1.24 - Treacher Collins syndrome

II. Treacher Collins Syndrome

   A. Derangement of the 1st and 2nd pharyngeal arches

   B. Autosomal dominant disorder

   C. Associated with neural crest cell dysfunction

   D. Facial abnormalities (eg, mandibular and zygomatic bone hypoplasia)

   E. Airway compromise

   F. Hearing loss

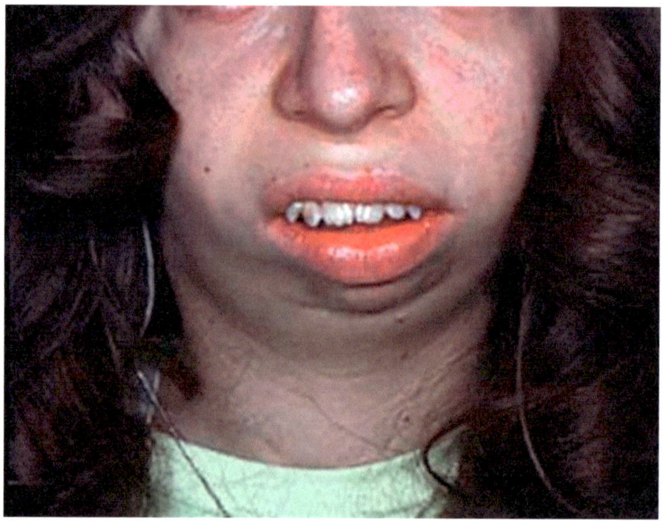

Photo Credit: Elements of morphology, National Human Genome Research Institute

Figure 6.1.25 - Pierre Robin sequence

III. Pierre Robin sequence

   A. Derangement of the 1st and 2nd pharyngeal arches

   B. Micrognathia

   C. Cleft palate

      1. Glossoptosis

      2. Airway obstruction

Section IX - 3rd, 4th and 6th Pharyngeal Arches

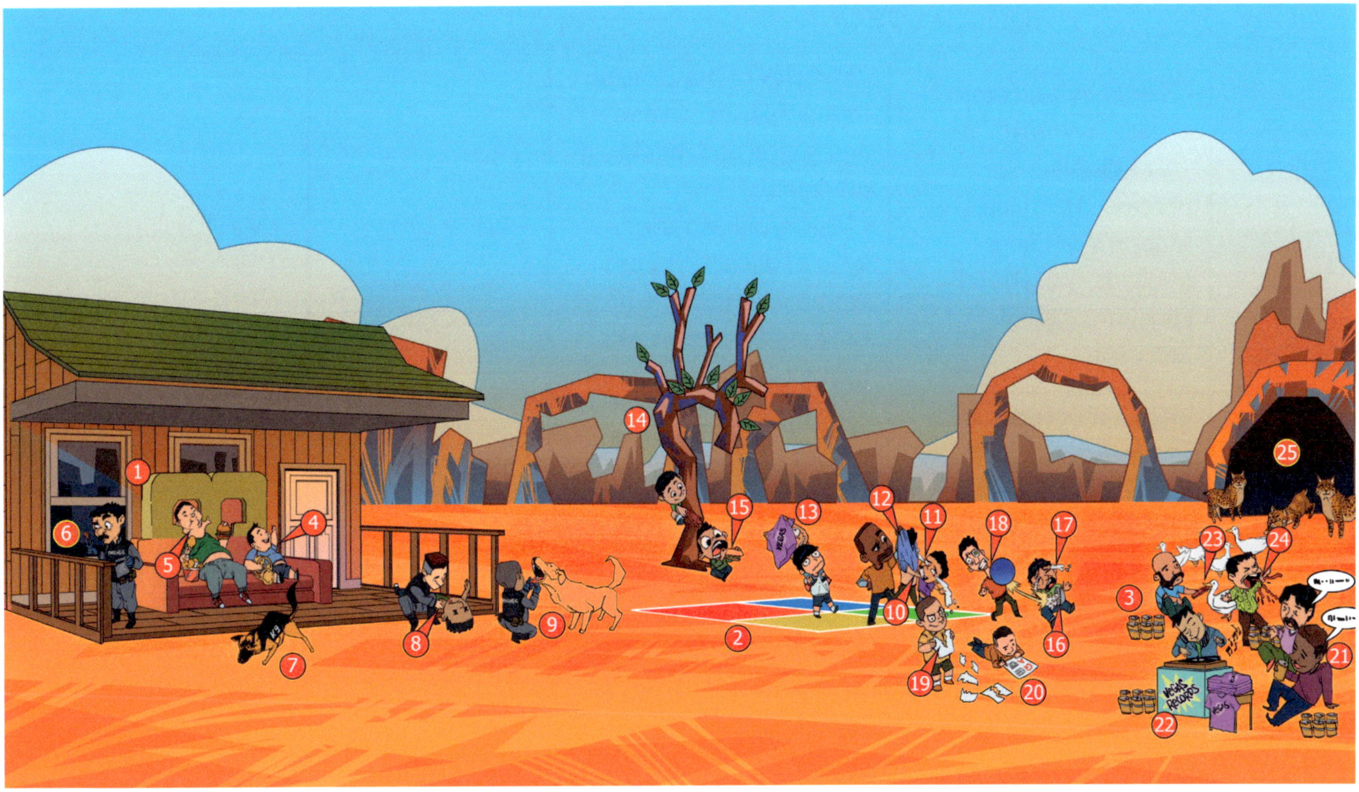

1. ____________________
2. ____________________
3. ____________________
4. ____________________
5. ____________________
6. ____________________
7. ____________________
8. ____________________
9. ____________________
10. ____________________
11. ____________________
12. ____________________
13. ____________________

Arch	Cartilage	Muscles	Nerves	Arteries
1st	- **Maxillary process**: maxilla, zygomatic bone - **Mandibular process**: mandible, Meckel's cartilage (malleus, incus), and sphenomandibular ligament	- **Muscles of mastication** (temporalis, masseter, and lateral and medial pterygoids) - Mylohyoid, anterior belly of digastric, tensor tympani, anterior ⅔ of tongue, and tensor veli palatini	- CN V_3	- Maxillary artery
2nd	- **Reichert's cartilage**: stapes, styloid, lesser horn of hyoid, stylohyoid ligament	- **Muscles of facial expression**: stapedius, stylohyoid, platysma, posterior belly of digastric	- CN VII	- Stapedial artery - Hyoid artery
3rd	- Greater horn of hyoid	- Stylopharyngeus - Posterior ⅓ of tongue	- CN IX	- Common carotid arteries - Proximal part of internal carotid
4th	- Arytenoids, cricoid, corniculate, cuneiform, and thyroid	- Cricothyroid, levator veli palatini, pharyngeal constrictors, and the posterior ⅓ of the tongue	- CN X (superior laryngeal branch)	- Left: aortic arch - Right: proximal part of subclavian artery
6th		- Intrinsic muscles of larynx (except cricothyroid)	- CN X (inferior laryngeal branch)	- Proximal part of pulmonary arteries - Ductus arteriosus

Table 6.1.6 - Pharyngeal arches

REVIEW QUESTIONS

1. A medical student is being tested on the cranial nerves in a gross anatomy laboratory. A nerve is pinned that is associated with taste and sensation of the posterior ⅓ of the tongue. The pharyngeal arch associated with this nerve gives rise to which of the following structures?

   A. Stylohyoid muscle
   B. Mylohyoid muscle
   C. Levator veli palatini muscle
   D. Stylopharyngeus muscle

- **Choice D is the correct answer.**
- **The cranial nerve being described is the glossopharyngeal nerve, or cranial nerve 9. Only the glossopharyngeal nerve is associated with taste and sensation of the posterior ⅓ of the tongue.**
- **The 9th cranial nerve is also associated with the 3rd pharyngeal arch which gives rise to the stylopharyngeus muscle so choice D is the correct answer.**
- **A is incorrect because this develops from the second pharyngeal arch.**
- **B is incorrect because it develops from the first pharyngeal arch.**
- **C is incorrect because it's developed from the 4th pharyngeal arch.**

Section X - Cleft Lip and Palate

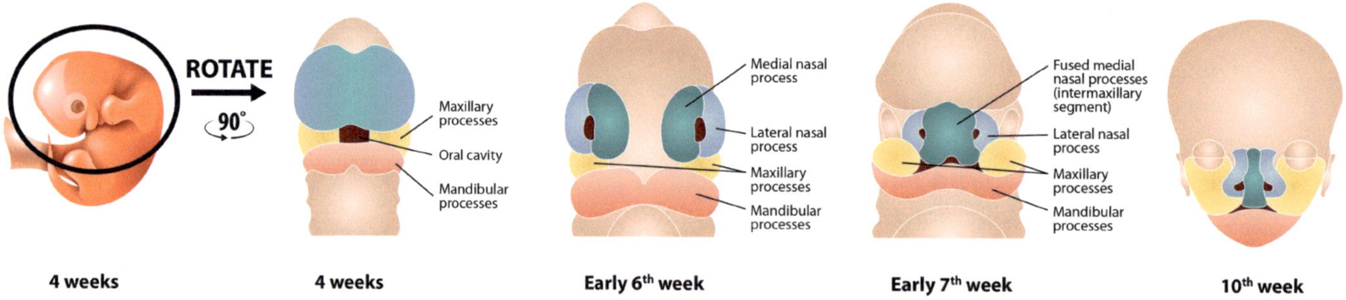

Figure 6.1.26 - Fetal facial development

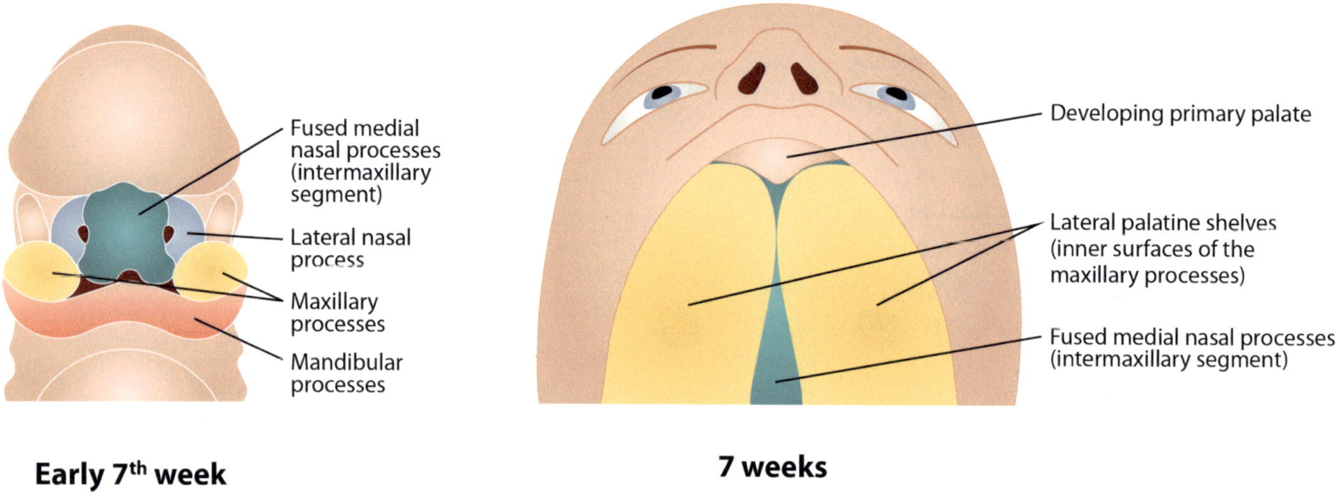

Figure 6.1.27 - Primary palate development

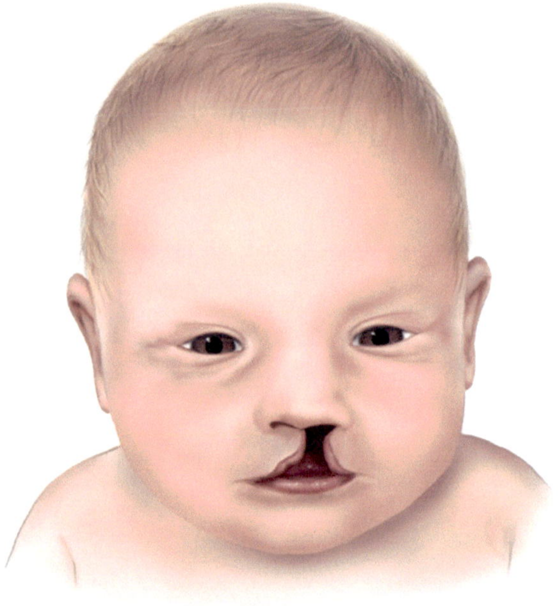

Photo Credit: Centers for Disease Control and Prevention

Figure 6.1.28 - Cleft lip

I. Cleft Lip
   A. Congenital birth defect
   B. Due to failure of the primary palate to form
   C. The primary palate forms as the maxillary processes fuse with the merged medial nasal processes (intermaxillary segment)
   D. Etiology is multifactorial (eg, genetic, environmental)
   E. Often occurs with cleft palate

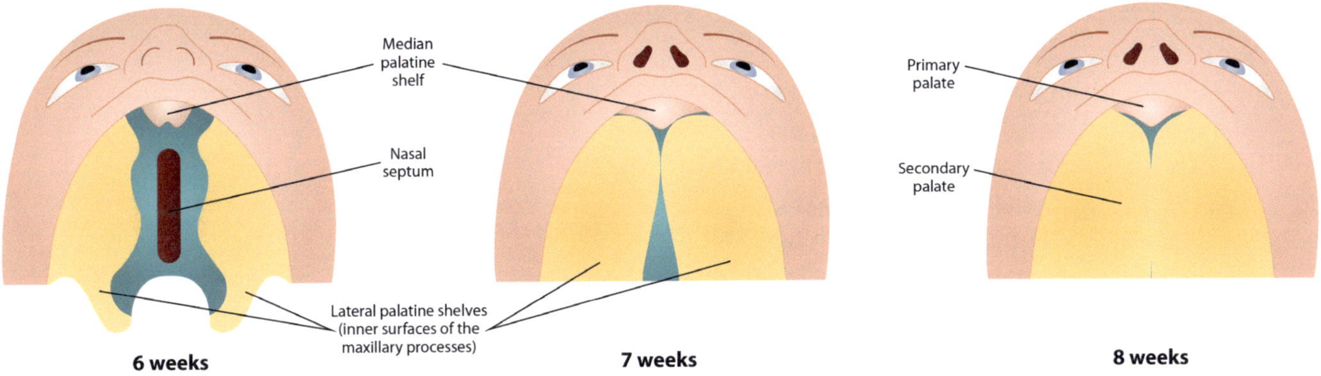

Figure 6.1.29 - Secondary palate development

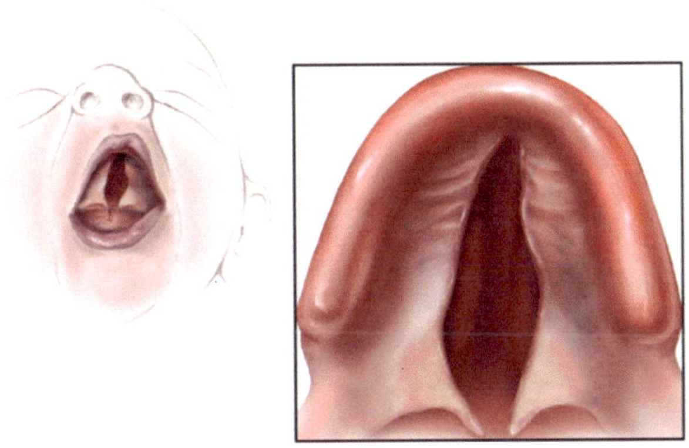

Photo Credit: Klem [CC BY 3.0 (https://creativecommons.org/licenses/by/3.0)]

Figure 6.1.30 - Cleft palate

I. Cleft Palate

A. Congenital birth defect

B. Due to failure of the secondary palate to form

C. The secondary palate forms as the lateral palatine shelves fuse together, with the nasal septum, and with the median palatine shelf

D. Etiology is multifactorial (eg, genetic, environmental)

E. Often occurs with cleft lip

REVIEW QUESTIONS

1. A 21-year-old pregnant female presents to the physician for an ultrasound during the second trimester of pregnancy. After thorough evaluation, the mother is informed that her child may have a cleft lip. If the child is born with a cleft lip, what process will have failed to fuse with the intermaxillary segment?

   A. Frontonasal
   B. Lateral
   C. Mandibular
   D. Maxillary

- **The correct choice is D.**
- **The fetus likely has a cleft lip discovered on ultrasound.**
- **Cleft lips are due to failure of fusion of the intermaxillary segment and the maxillary process.**
- **The fused medial nasal processes, or intermaxillary segment, fuse with the maxillary processes to form the primary palate.**
- **A is incorrect because the intermaxillary segment doesn't fuse with the frontonasal process. The frontonasal process is associated with the forehead.**
- **B is incorrect because failure of fusion of the lateral palatine shelves is associated with a cleft palate - not a cleft lip**
- **C is incorrect because the mandibular processes fuse together to form the lower part of the jaw including the mandible.**

Section XI - Normal Genital Development

I. Overview

A. Genetic sex (XY or XX) is determined at conception

B. Gonads (testes or ovaries) determined by SRY gene

1. Default development → female
2. SRY gene on the Y chromosome → male

C. Internal and external genitalia determined by hormones

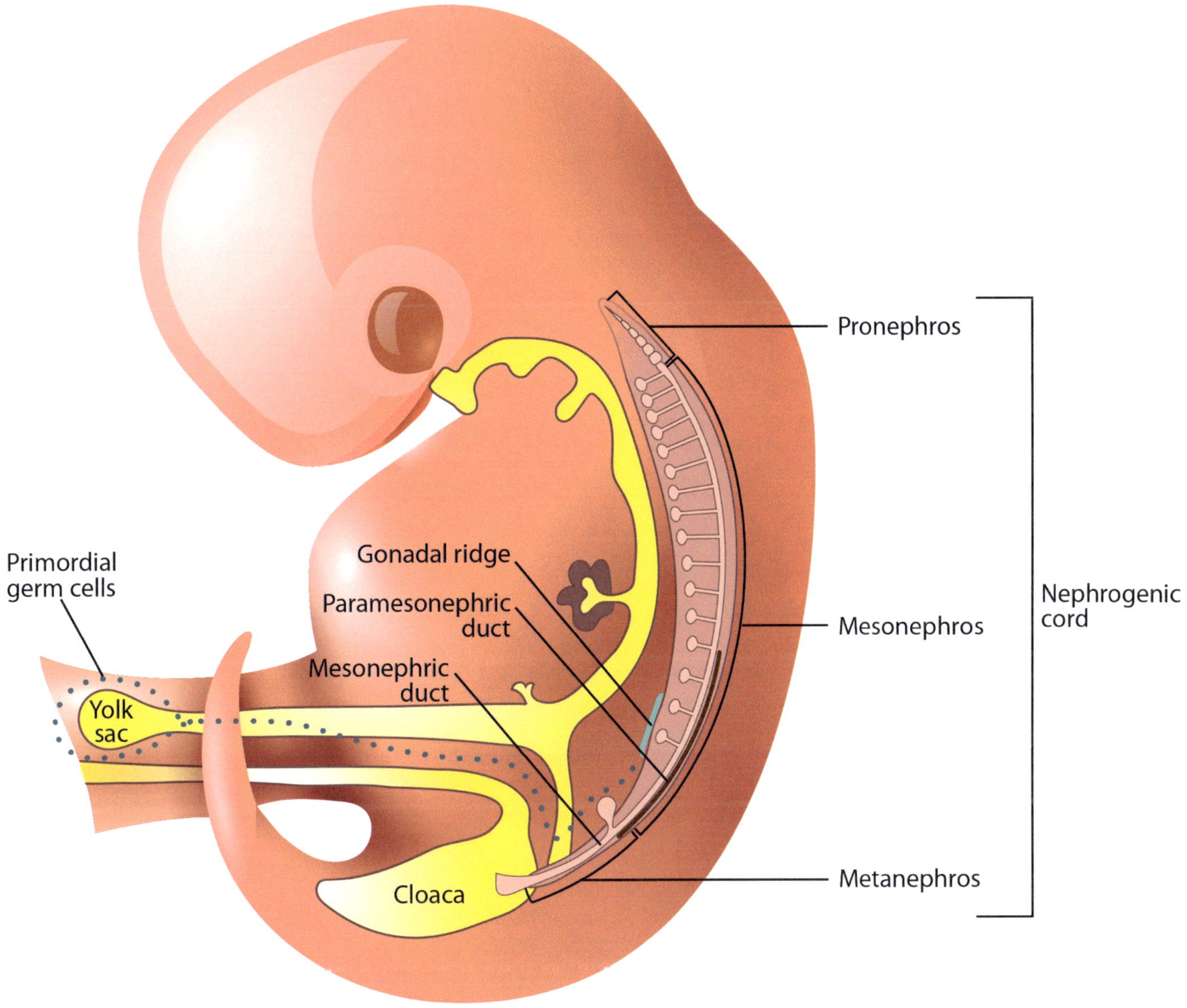

Figure 6.1.31 - Lateral view of the nephrogenic cord

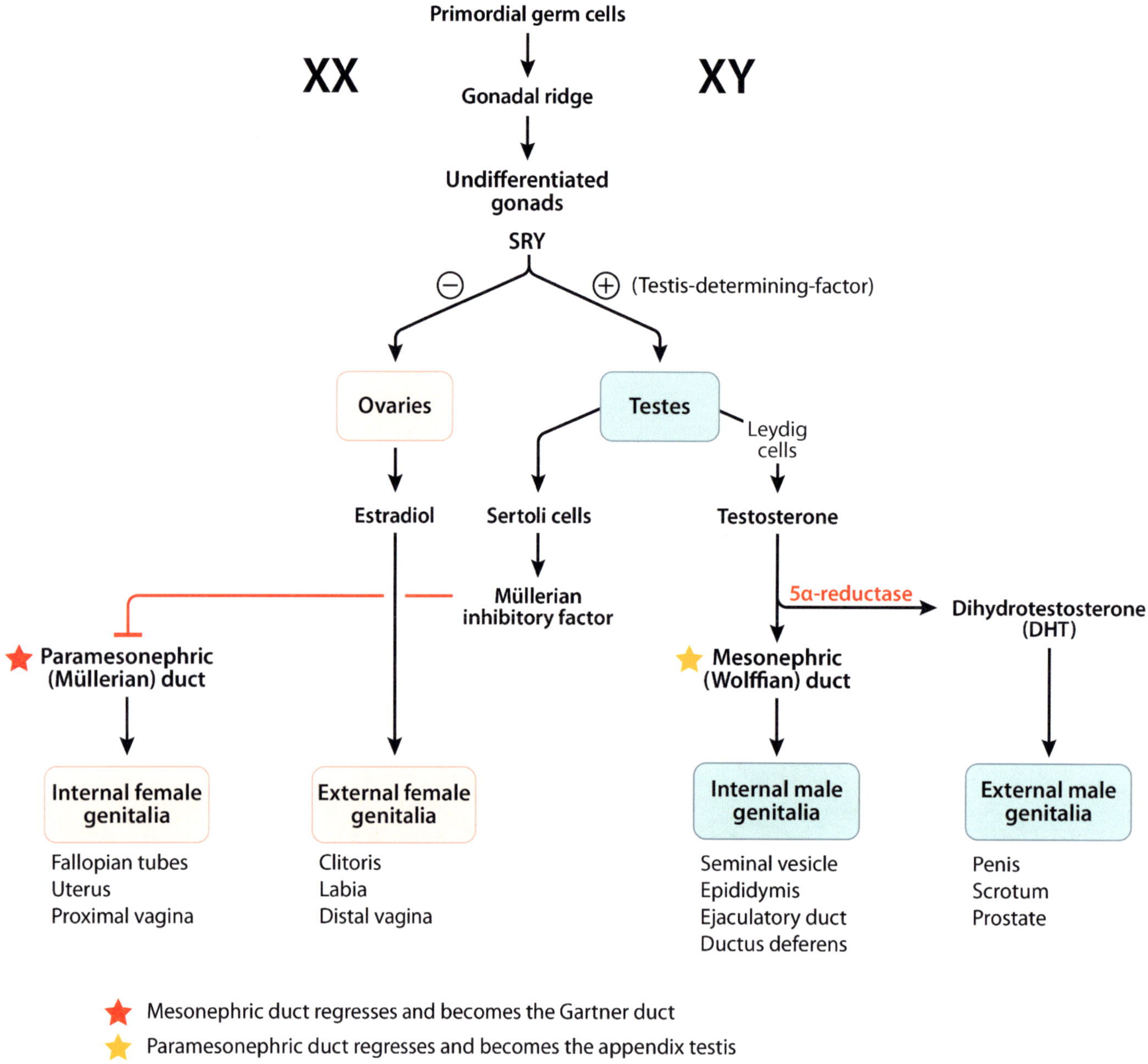

Figure 6.1.32 - Male and female sexual differentiation overview

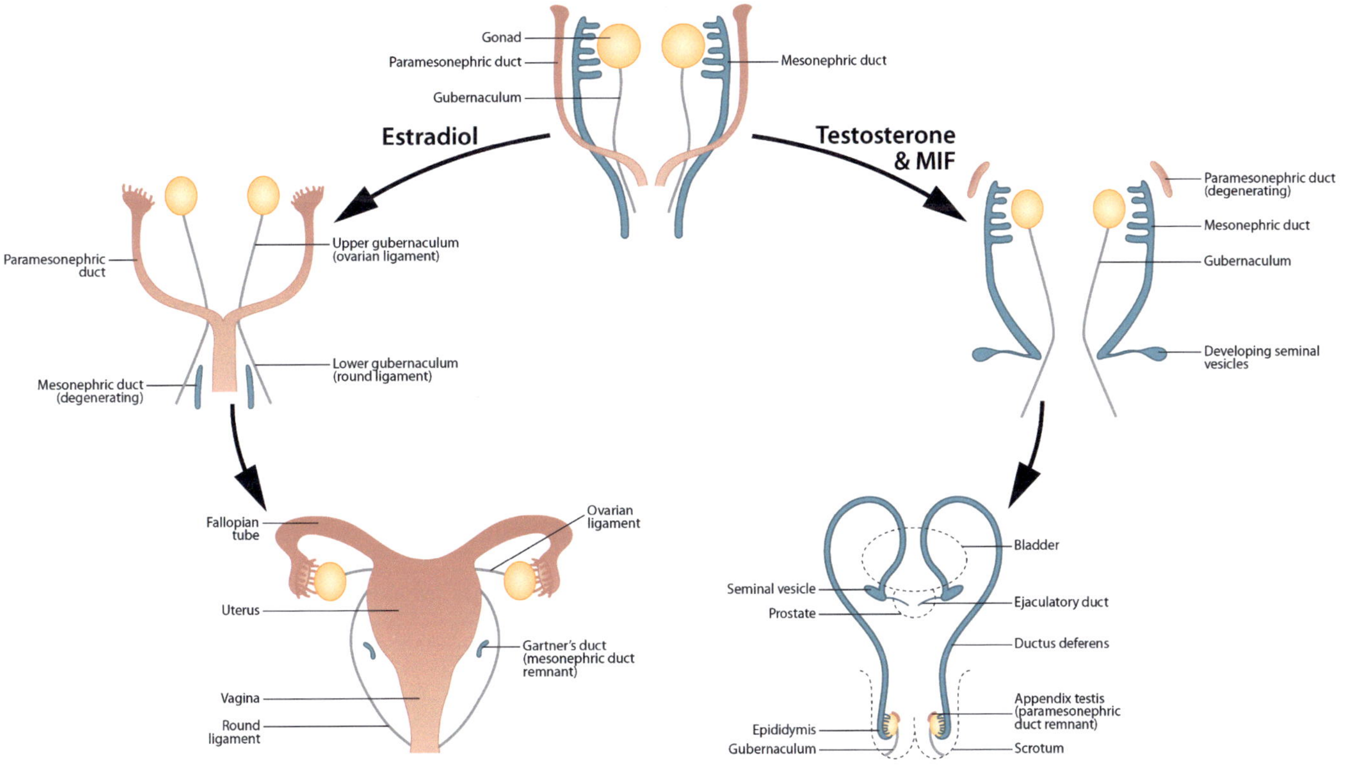

Figure 6.1.33 - Undifferentiated gonadal development

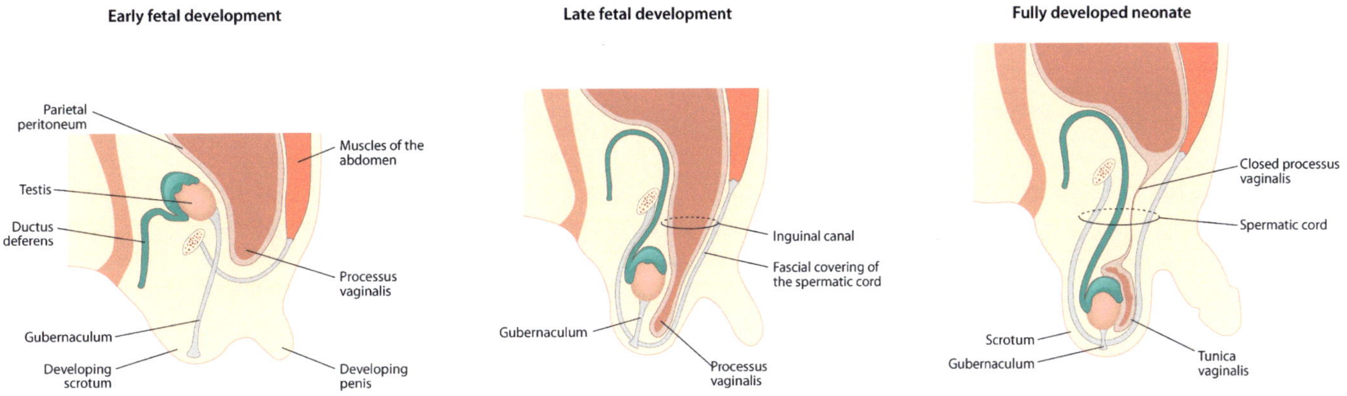

Figure 6.1.34 - Gonadal descent

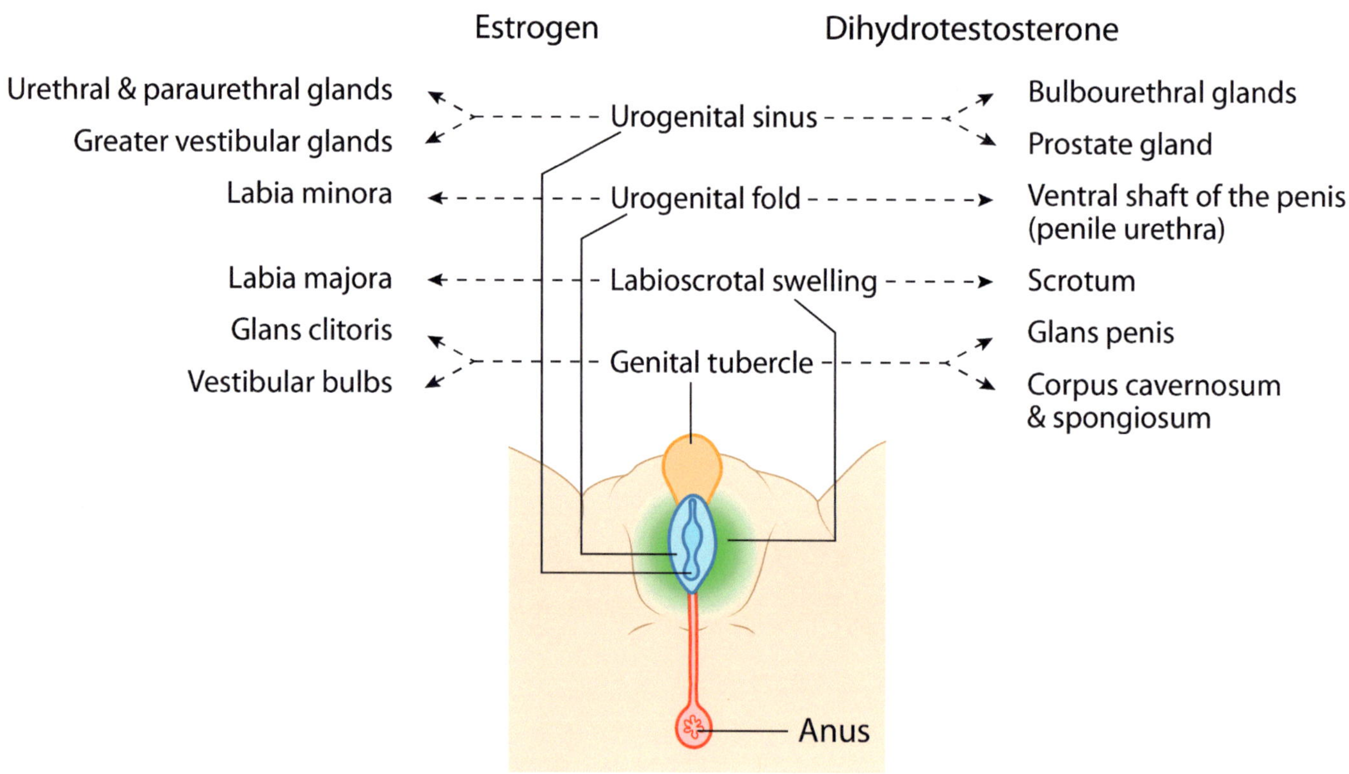

Figure 6.1.35 - External genitalia differentiation

REVIEW QUESTIONS

1. If the Sertoli cells in a male (XY) infant are dysfunctional, what internal genitalia will be expected to form?

   - **This male patient will have both internal female and internal male genitalia.**
   - **Sertoli cells produce müllerian inhibitory factor which normally results in degeneration of the paramesonephric duct.**
   - **If this is absent, then both the paramesonephric duct and the mesonephric duct will form.**
   - **The sertoli cells normally produce müllerian inhibitory factor which causes degeneration of the paramesonephric duct.**
   - **If this is absent, then the paramesonephric duct won't degenerate, and this male will end up developing internal female genitalia along with internal male genitalia.**

Section XII - Pathology of Genital Development

I. Overview

   A. Müllerian agenesis

   B. Uterine anomalies

   C. MIF-related disorders

   D. 5α-reductase deficiency

   E. Congenital penile abnormalities

II. Müllerian Agenesis (Mayer-Rokitansky-Küster-Hauser Syndrome)

   A. Due to hypoplasia or agenesis of the paramesonephric duct (Müllerian duct) → internal genitalia defect (eg, vagina, uterus)

   B. Etiology not well understood

   C. Presentation:

      1. Phenotypically female

      2. Genetic sex is XX

      3. Primary amenorrhea (uterine defect)

      4. Fully developed secondary sexual characteristics (ovaries present)

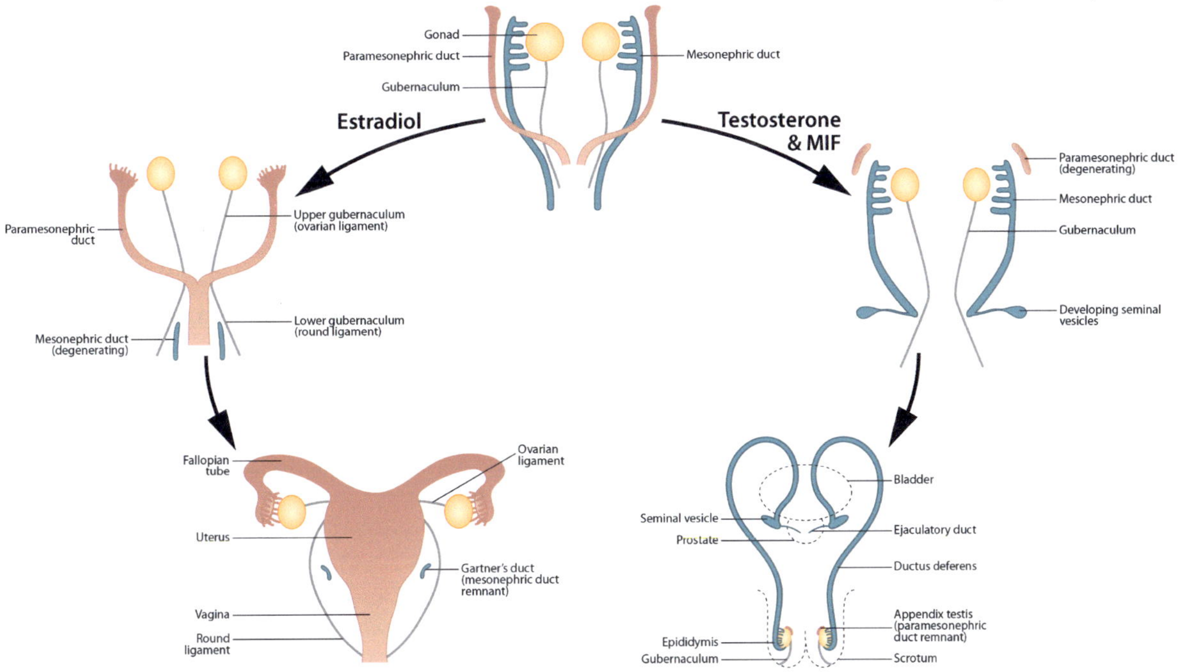

Figure 6.1.33 - Undifferentiated gonadal development

Uterine anomaly	Etiology	Findings	Other
Septate uterus	- Failed resorption of the septum between the fused paramesonephric ducts	- Indented endometrial cavity with a smooth fundus	- ↑ risk of pregnancy complications - Treat with septoplasty
Bicornuate uterus	- Incomplete fusion of the paramesonephric ducts	- Indented fundus of the uterus (cervix and vagina are normal) - Uterine horns may be completely, partially, or only minimally separated	- ↑ risk of pregnancy complications
Uterus didelphys	- Complete failure of the paramesonephric ducts to fuse	- Double vagina, cervix, and uterus	- ↑ risk of pregnancy complications (pregnancy is possible)

Table 6.1.7 - Uterine anomalies

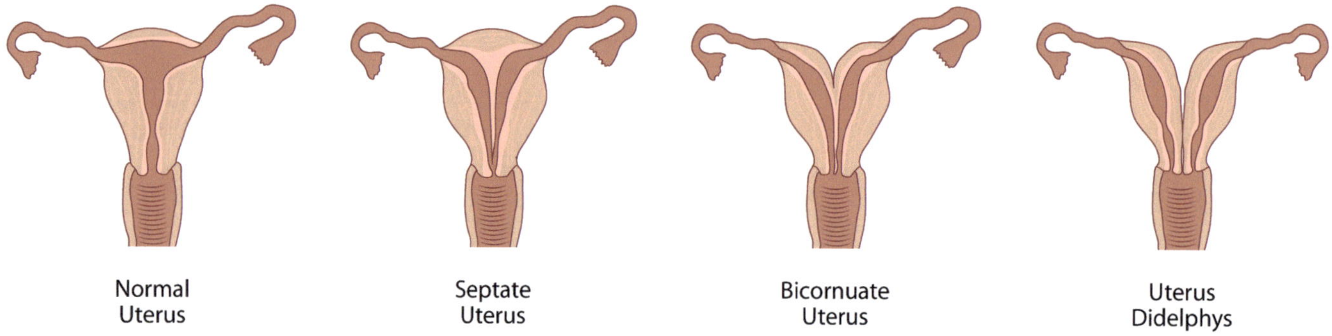

Figure 6.1.36 - Uterine anomalies

III. MIF-related Disorders

A. ↓ Müllerian inhibitory factor (MIF) → internal female genitalia persist

B. Karyotype of MIF-related disorders is 46, XY

C. Phenotype is male

D. Three causes:

1. Absence of Sertoli cells
2. Lack of MIF
3. Persistent Müllerian duct syndrome
    a) Defect in anti-Müllerian hormone (AMH) gene
    b) Undescended testes and an inguinal hernia

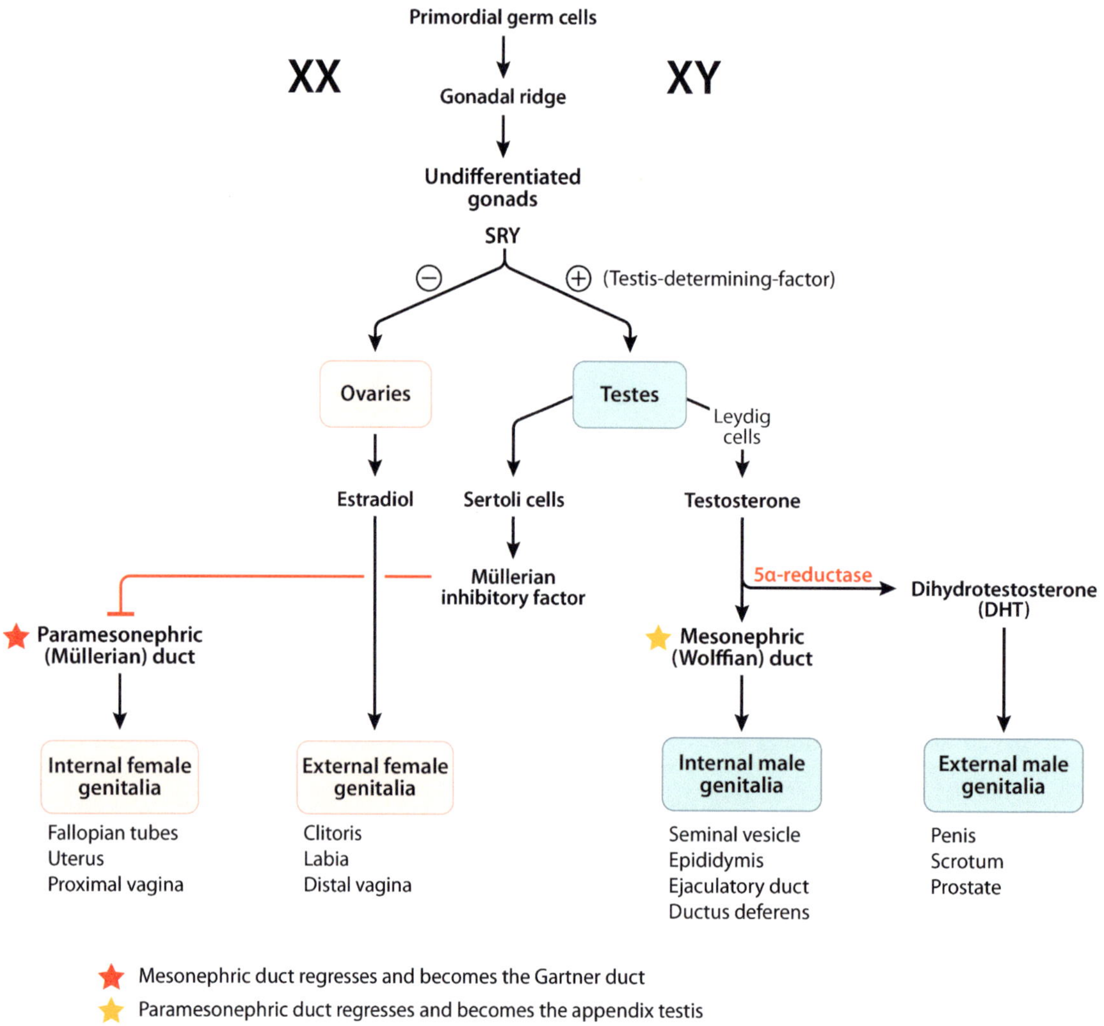

Figure 6.1.32 - Male and female sexual differentiation overview

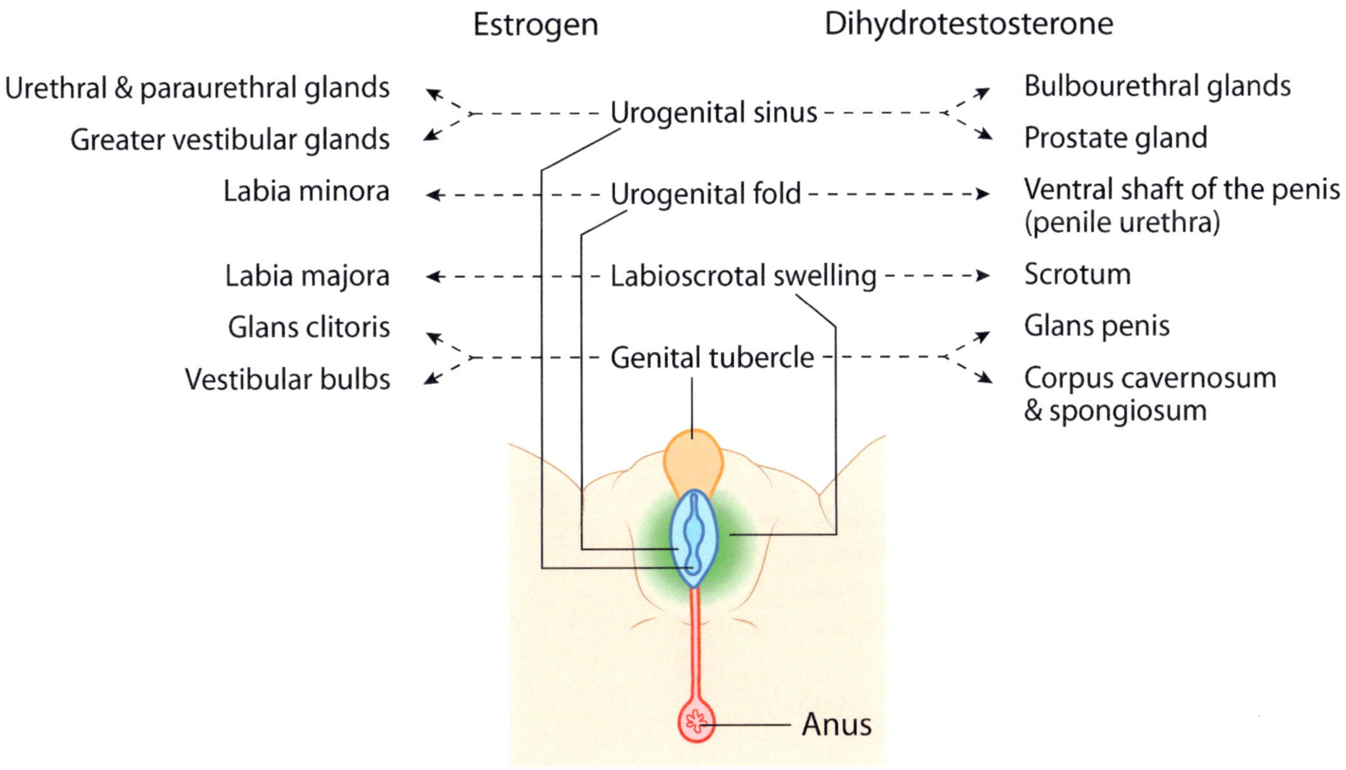

Figure 6.1.35 - External genitalia differentiation

IV. 5α-reductase Deficiency

A. 5α-reductase converts testosterone → DHT

B. DHT is necessary for the development of the external male genitalia

C. Deficiency

1. Karyotype is typically 46, XY
2. Normal internal male genitalia
3. External female genitalia (may be ambiguous) at birth
4. At puberty testosterone level rise → normal male genitalia

V. Congenital Penile Abnormalities

A. Epispadias

1. Genital tubercle migrates abnormally
2. Opening of the urethra on the dorsal surface (top)
3. Epispadias → pEE in your Eye
4. Associated with bladder exstrophy

B. Hypospadias (more common)

1. Failure of the urethral folds to fuse on the ventral surface (bottom)
2. Associated with inguinal hernias, cryptorchidism, and chordee

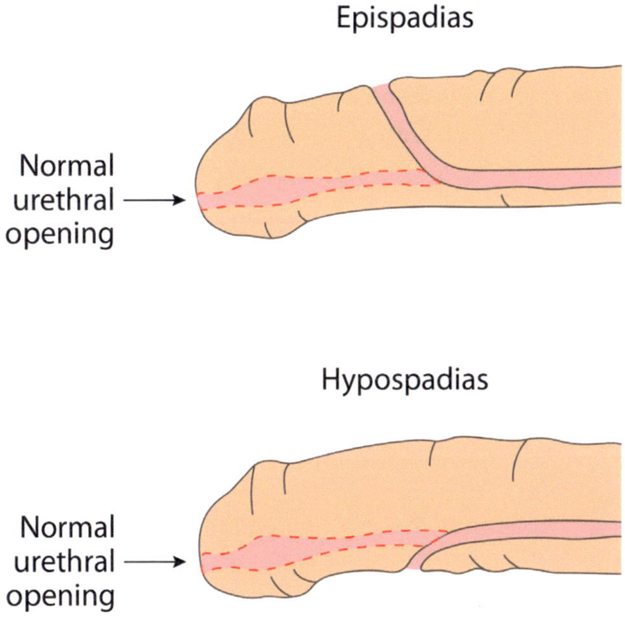

Figure 6.1.36 - Hypospadias and epispadias

REVIEW QUESTIONS ?

3. A newborn girl is found to have an enlarged clitoris but is otherwise normal. Her parents are concerned and decide to do genetic testing which reveals that the karyotype of their child is 46, XY. Further investigation reveals that this child's condition is due to an enzyme deficiency that normally produces a more potent form of testosterone. An abdominal ultrasound of the child will most likely reveal which type of genitalia?

- **Correct answer: internal male genitalia**
- **This child has an enlarged clitoris, a karyotype of 46, XY, and an enzyme deficiency that normally produces a more potent form of testosterone.**
- **Collectively, these clues should make you think of 5α-reductase deficiency.**
- **In this condition, a lack of testosterone during fetal development results in failure to adequately form the external male genitalia.**
- **The internal male genitalia form just fine.**
- **Therefore, an abdominal ultrasound will most likely reveal internal male genitalia.**
- **Recall that 5α-reductase normally converts testosterone to dihydrotestosterone and that this is responsible for the development of external male genitalia.**
- **Therefore if it's deficient, then the external male genitalia will not be formed at birth.**

CARDIOLOGY

Section I - Normal Cardiac Development

I. Overview

A. Embryonic precursors

B. Cardiac looping

C. Septation of the atria

D. Septation of the ventricles

E. Septation of the outflow tract

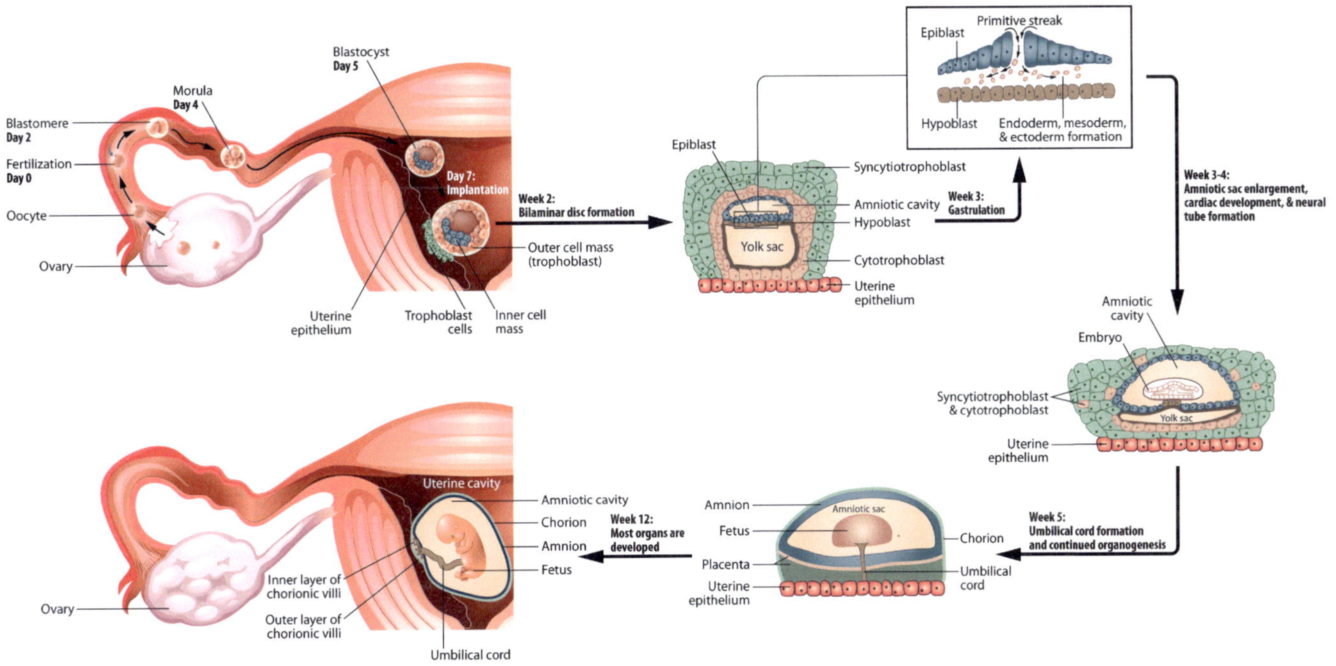

Figure 6.1.1 - Early fetal development

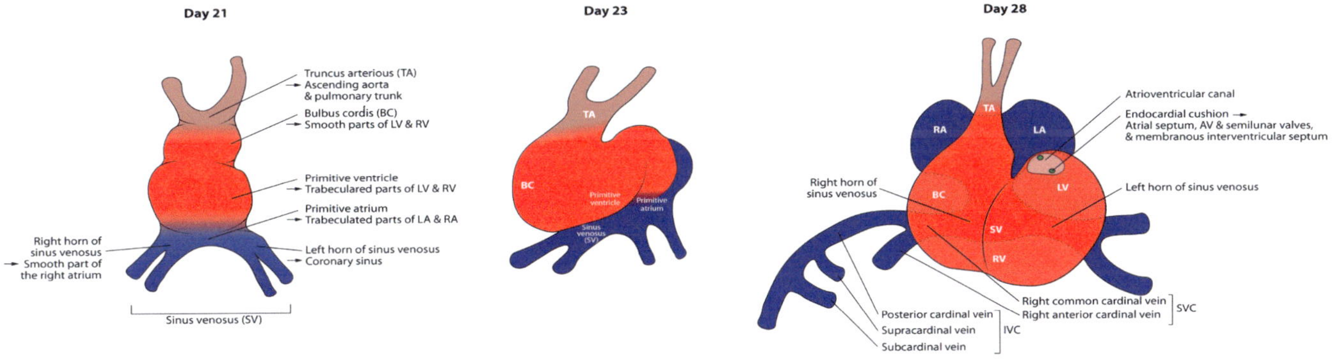

Figure 6.2.1 - Cardiac development around 3-4 weeks

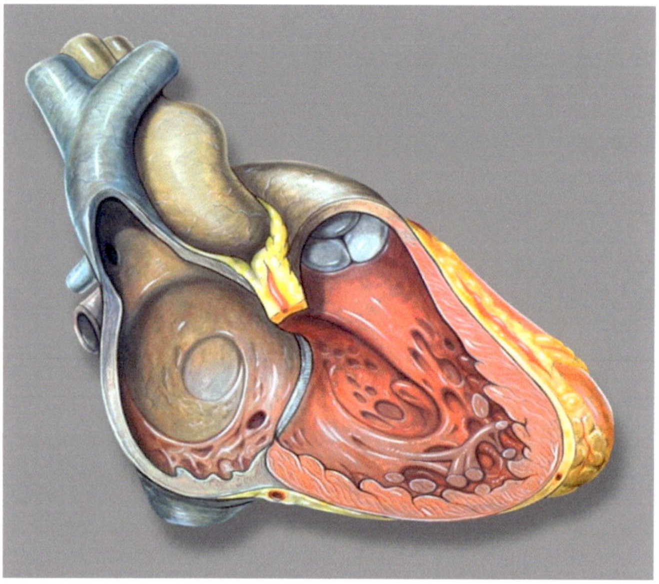

Figure 6.2.3 - Smooth and trabeculated regions of the heart

Embryonic Structure	Adult Structure
Truncus arteriosus	- Ascending aorta - Pulmonary trunk
Bulbus cordis	- Smooth portions of the left and right ventricles
Primitive ventricle	- Trabeculated portion of the left and right ventricle
Primitive atria	- Trabeculated portions of the left and right atria
Primitive pulmonary vein	- Smooth portion of the left atrium
Right horn of sinus venosus	- Smooth portion of the right atrium
Left horn of sinus venosus	- Coronary sinus
Right common cardinal vein	- Superior vena cava
Posterior, subcardinal, and supracardinal veins	- Inferior vena cava
Endocardial cushion	- Atrial septum - Membranous interventricular septum - AV and semilunar valves

Table 6.2.1 - Adult derivatives of embryonic structures

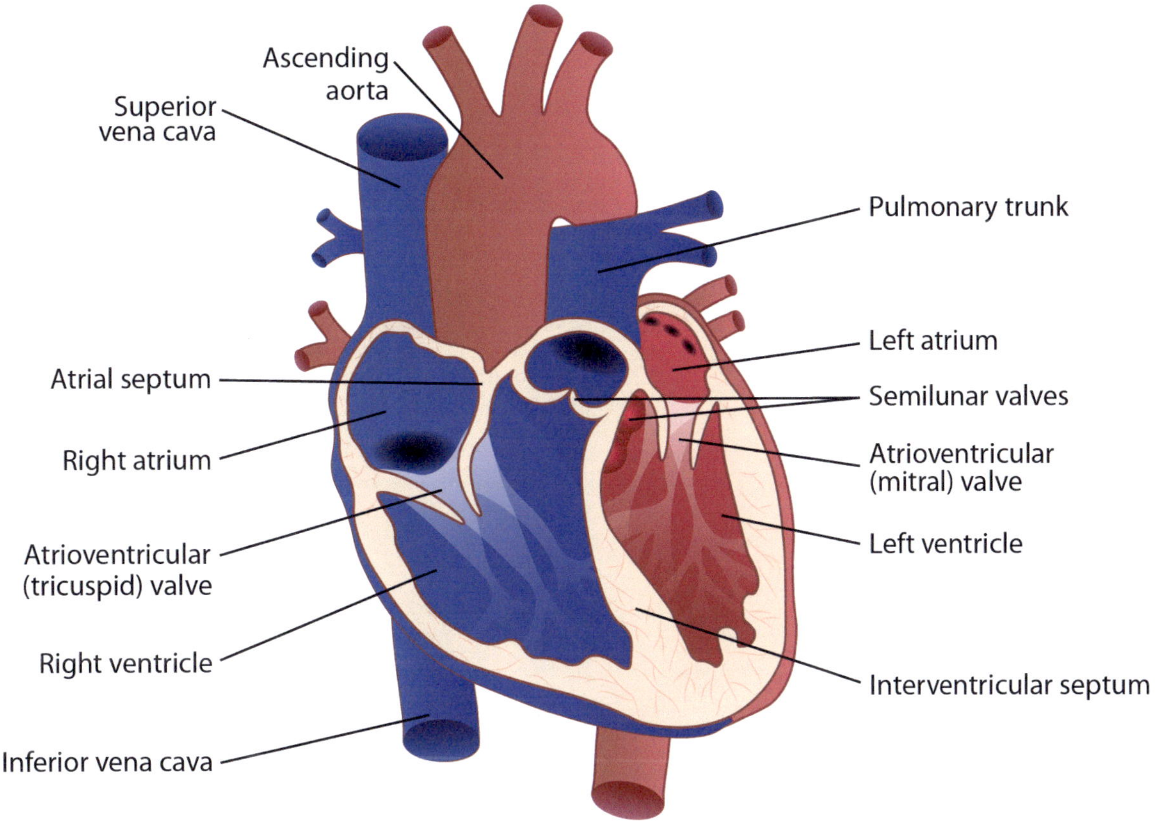

Figure 6.2.4 - Adult heart structures

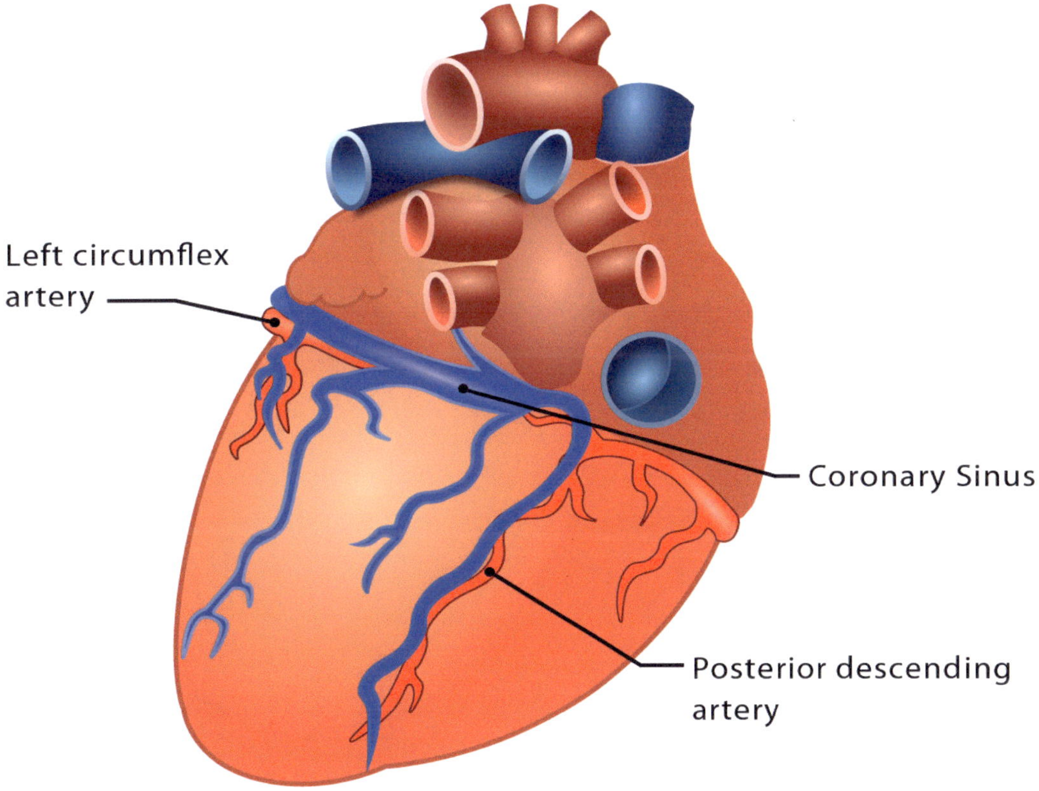

Figure 6.2.5 - Posterior view of the adult heart

II. Cardiac Looping

A. Helps establish the correct orientation of the heart

B. Begins during week 4 of gestation

a. Dynein defects can lead to dextrocardia (Kartagener syndrome)

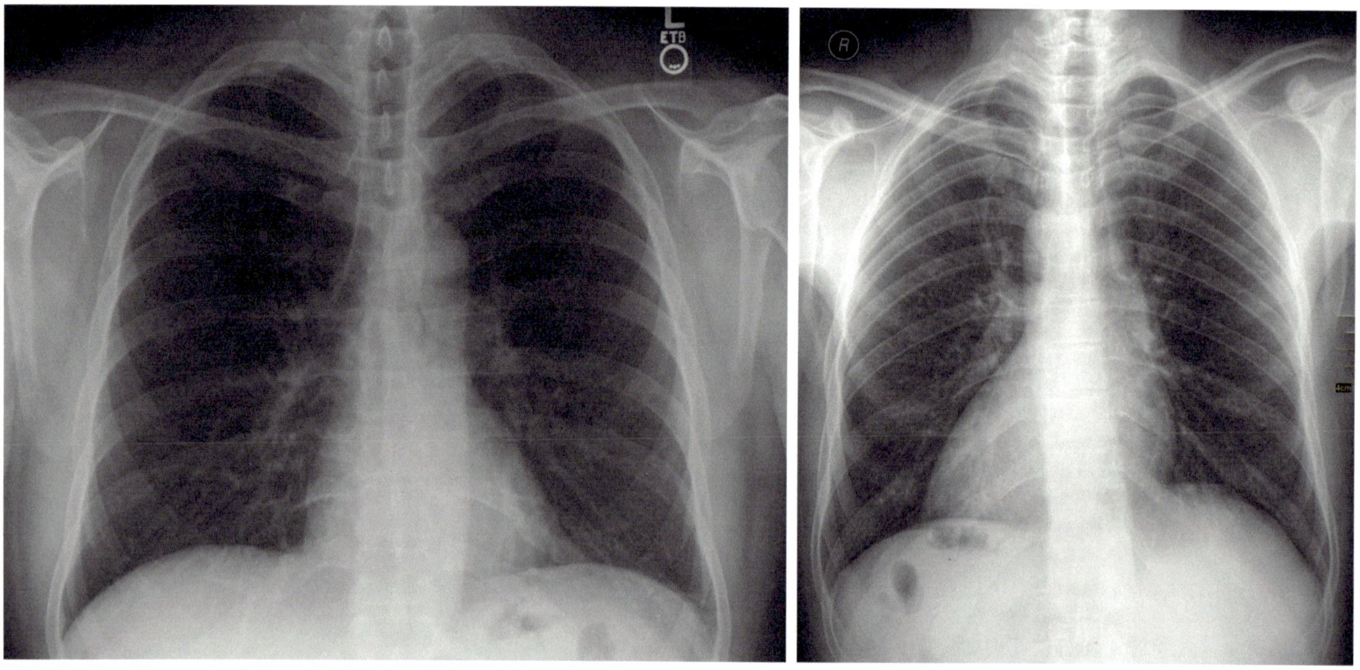

Photo Credit: Stillwaterising [CC0] (left), Nevit [CC BY-SA 3.0 (https://creativecommons.org/licenses/by-sa/3.0)] (right)

Figure 6.2.6 - Chest x-ray of heart (left: normal; right: dextrocardia)

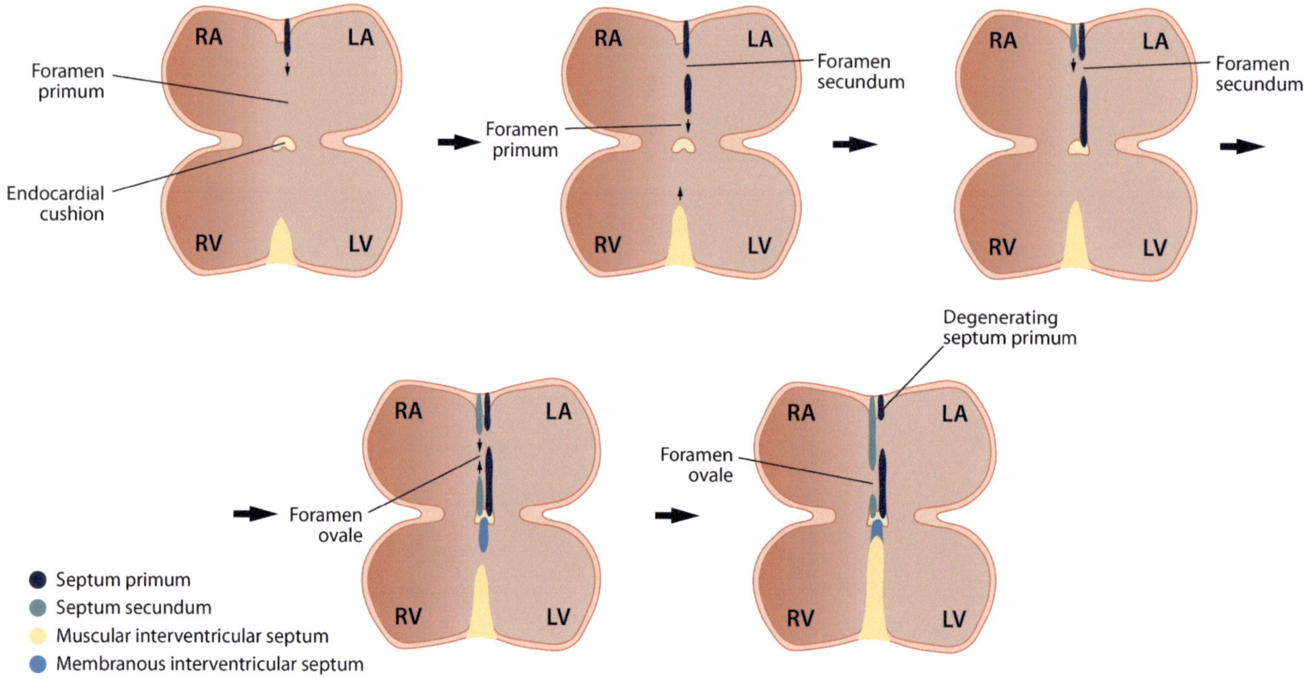

Figure 6.2.7 - Atrioventricular septae formation

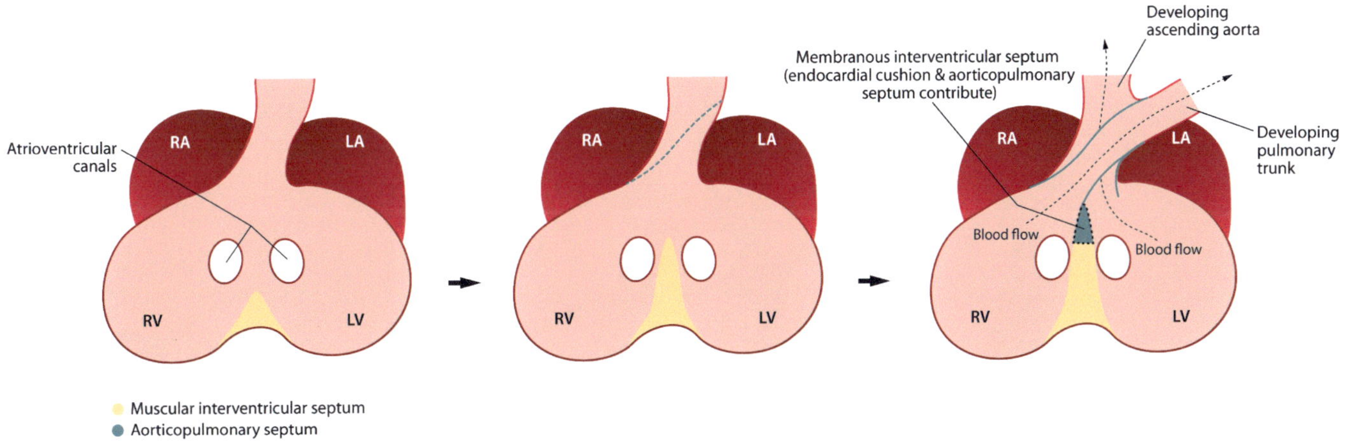

Figure 6.2.8 - Muscular interventricular septum and aorticopulmonary septum formation

REVIEW QUESTIONS

1. A newborn with a cardiac murmur is found to have a ventricular septal defect. The physician informs the parents that this most likely occurred due to failure of what embryological structure to develop properly?

   - **A VSD is most commonly due to failure of the membranous portion of the interventricular septum to develop properly.**
   - **Less frequently, failure of the muscular portion of the interventricular septum to develop properly can result in a VSD**

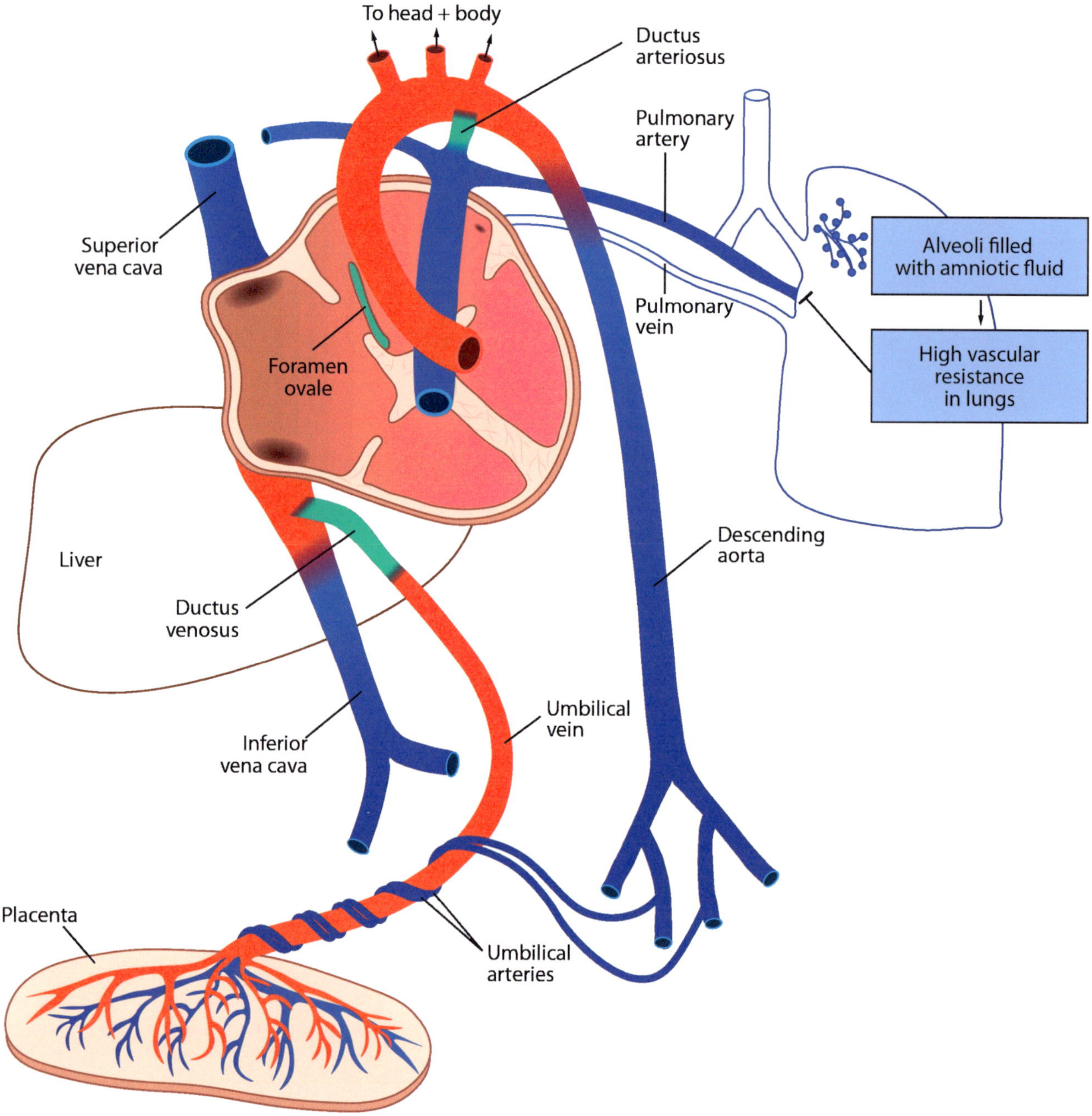

Figure 6.2.9 - Fetal circulation

I. Umbilical Vein

A. Carries oxygenated blood from the mother to the fetus

1. $Po_2 \approx$ 30 mmHg (after birth ≈ 100 mmHg)

2. 80% O_2 saturation (after birth ≈ 94-100%)

B. Drains into the IVC through the ductus venosus

C. Degenerates to become the ligamentum teres hepatis (round ligament)

II. Umbilical Arteries

A. Two vessels that carry deoxygenated blood from the fetus to the mother → low O_2 saturation

B. Drains blood from fetal internal iliac arteries

C. Degenerates to become the medial umbilical ligaments

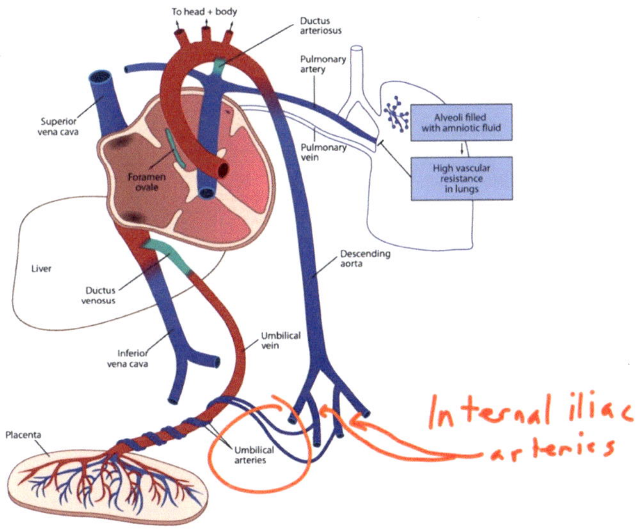

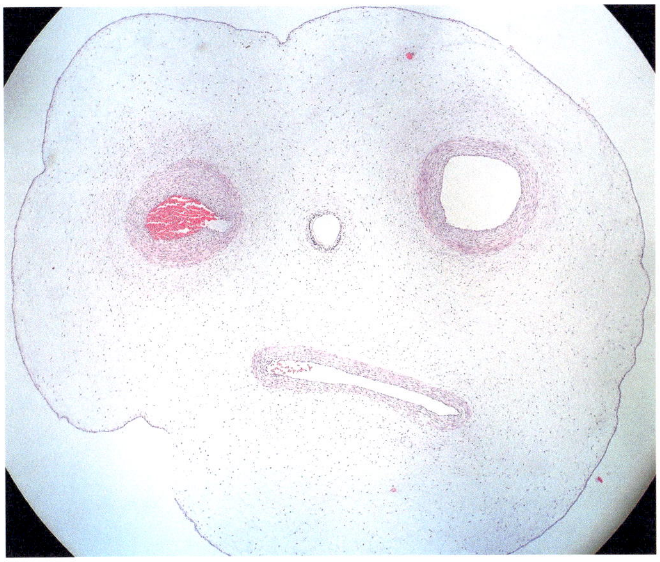

Photo Credit: Ed Uthman via Flickr (CC BY 2.0)

Figure 6.2.10 - Cross-sectional cut of the umbilical cord

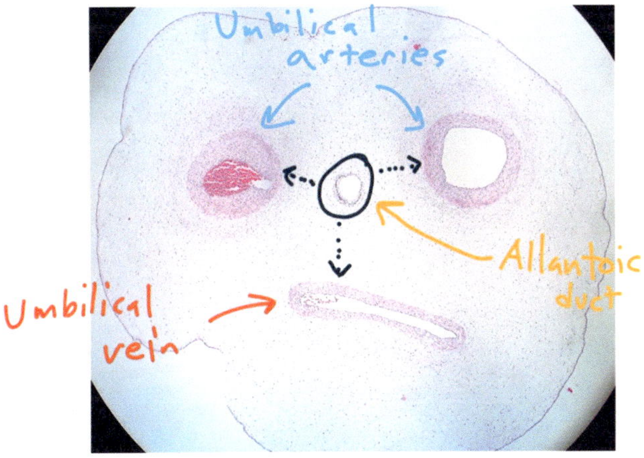

Ed Uthman via Flickr (CC BY 2.0)

III. Allantois

A. Connects bladder and umbilical cord

B. Drains fetal urine in the first trimester

C. Walls become umbilical vein and arteries

D. Obliterates to become the urachus → median umbilical ligament in adults

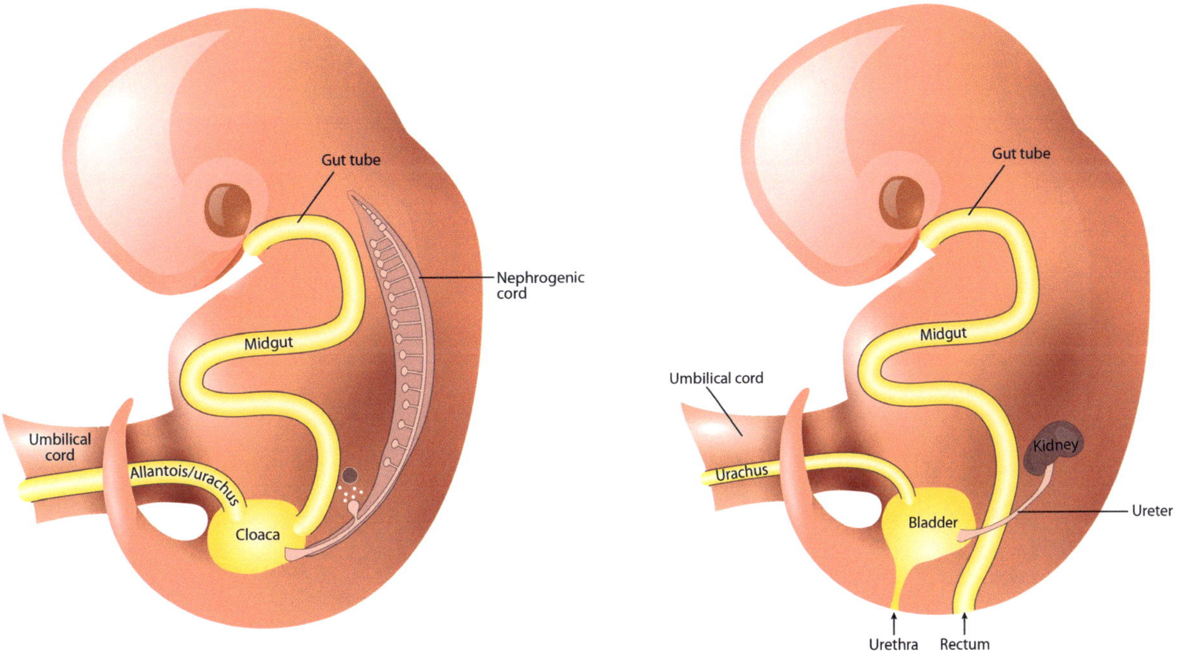

Figure 6.2.11 - Urinary excretion in 1st trimester (left), Urinary excretion in 2nd and 3rd trimesters (right)

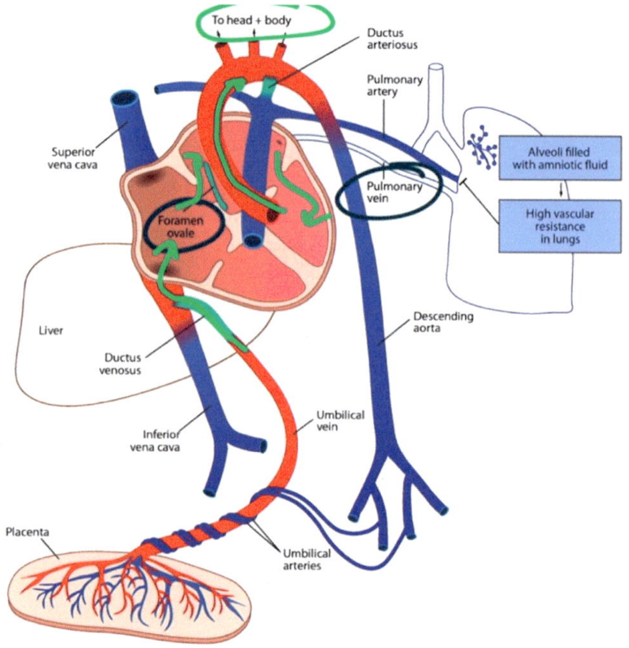

IV. Fetal Circulation

A. Umbilical vein → ductus venosus (bypasses liver) → inferior vena cava → right atrium → foramen ovale → left atrium → left ventricle → aorta → head and body

B. Right ventricle (when blood enters here) → pulmonary arteries → ductus arteriosus → aortic arch

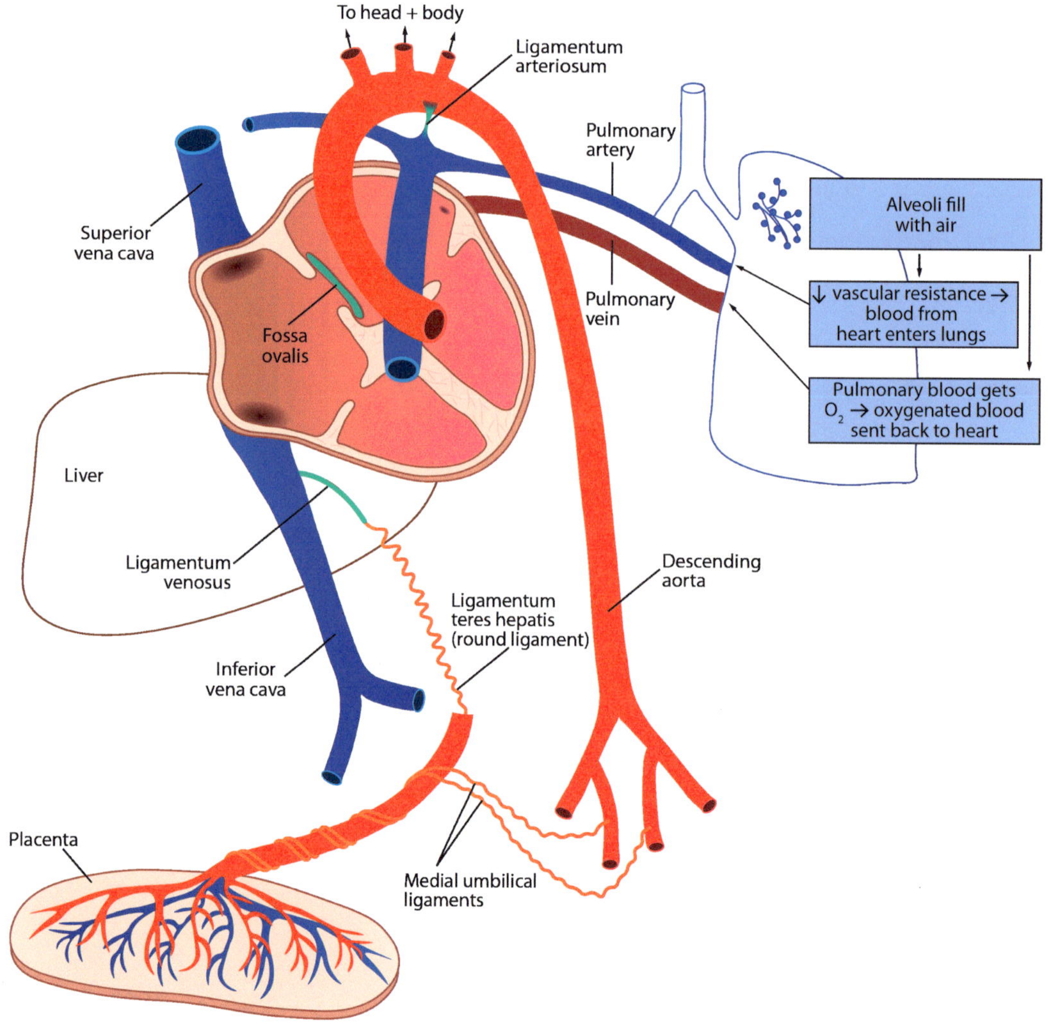

Figure 6.2.12 - Neonatal circulation

V. Neonatal Circulation

A. Blood enters right atrium from SVC and IVC → foramen ovale becomes fossa ovalis → blood travels from right atrium → right ventricle → pulmonary arteries (ductus arteriosus becomes ligamentum arteriosum) → pulmonary veins → left atrium → left ventricle → aorta → head and body

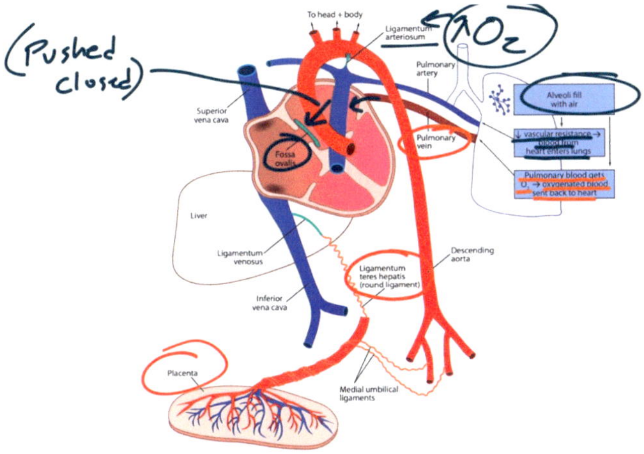

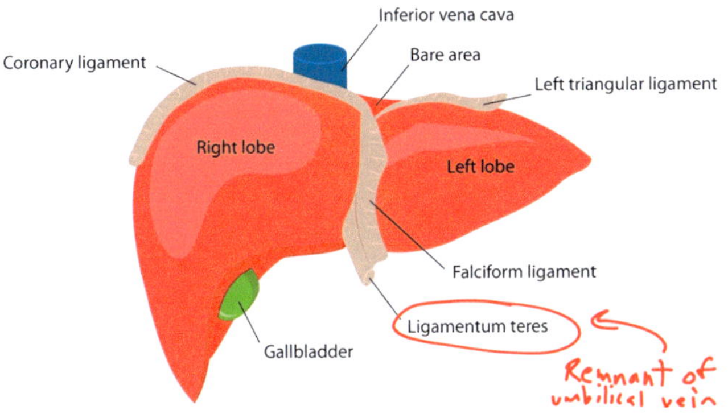

VI. Closing the Ductus Arteriosus

A. Breathing begins → ↑ O_2 (from 30 mmHg before to 100 mmHg after)

B. Placenta removed → ↓ prostaglandins (E_1 & E_2)

C. ↑ O_2 and ↓ PGE_1 & PGE_2 → ductus arteriosus closes (ligamentum arteriosum)

1. Prostaglandins - patency
2. Indomethacin - close

VII. Coarctation of the Aorta

A. Aortic narrowing near the ductus arteriosus/ ligamentum arteriosum

B. Congenital (70% of cases)

C. Acquired (30% of cases)

D. Congenital (70% of cases)

1. Associated with Turner syndrome and unclear genetic factors
2. Higher pressure proximal to coarctation → upper extremity hypertension, lower extremity hypotension (>10 mmHg difference)
3. Delayed, weak pulse in the lower extremities → brachial-femoral delay
4. Heart and vasculature cannot adapt quickly enough → CHF

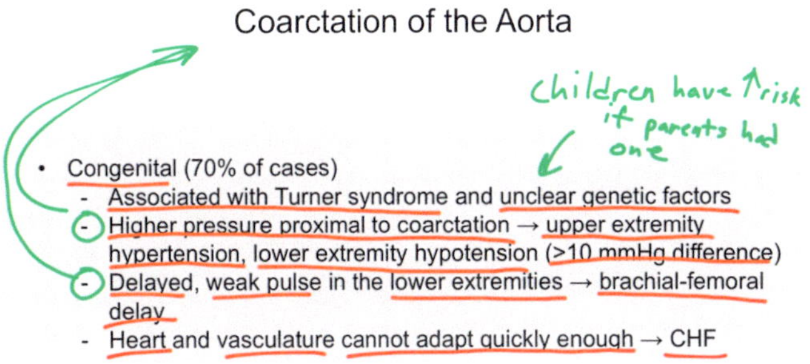

E. Acquired (30% of cases)

1. Mechanism unclear, but often occurs with bicuspid aortic valve
2. Brachial-femoral delay and >10 mmHg upper-lower limb difference (similar to congenital type)
3. Collateral circulations (retrograde flow from posterior to anterior intercostal arteries) → engorgement → rib notching on x-ray
4. Low blood flow to lower limbs → claudication
5. Increased pressure in cranial arteries → berry aneurysms

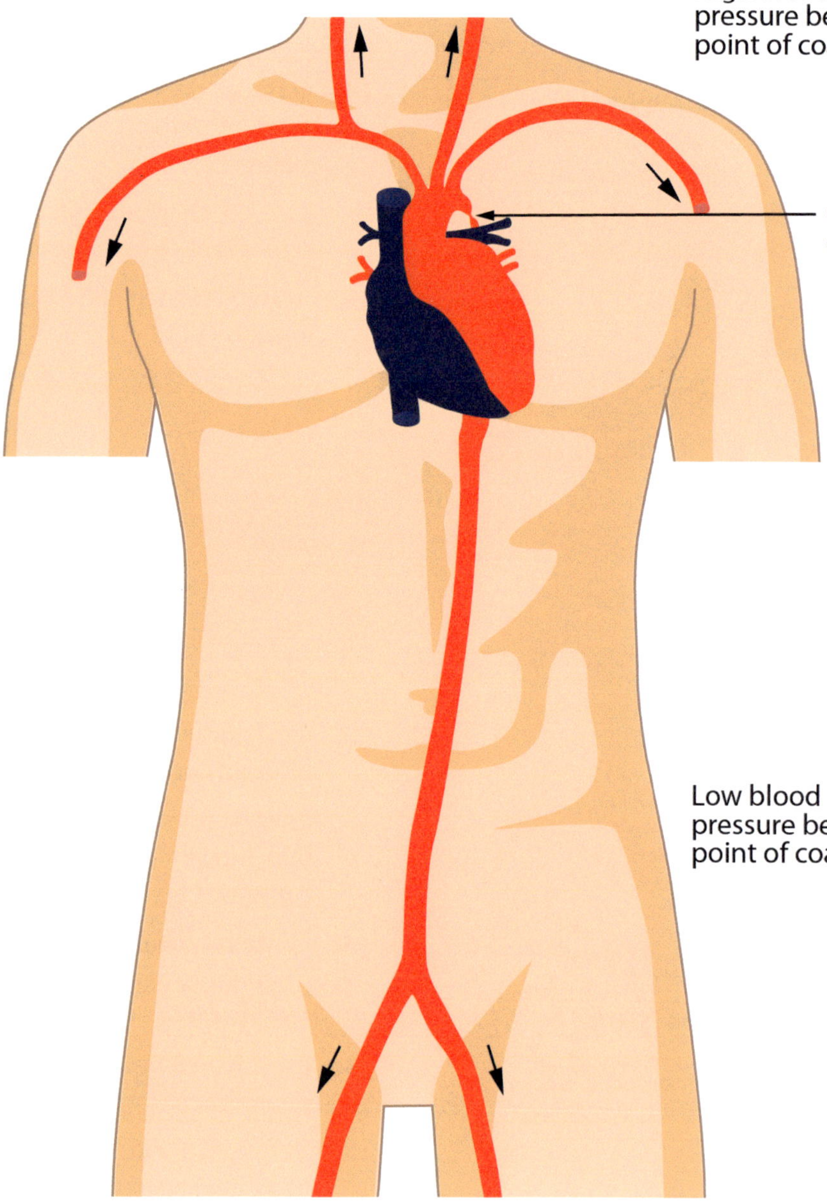

Figure 6.2.13 - Coarctation of the aorta

REVIEW QUESTIONS

1. Shortly after delivering a newborn, a physician examines contents of the umbilical cord and identifies a structure that typically has a $PO_{2,}$ around 30 mmHg in utero. Part of this structure remains in the newborn and will degenerate into what structure?

- **The structure described here is the umbilical vein.**
- **This is what carries oxygenated blood from the mother to the fetus and the partial pressure of oxygen in the umbilical vein is around 30 mmHg.**
- **The umbilical vein will degenerate into the ligamentum teres hepatis, part of the round ligament of the liver.**

Section III - Right-to-Left Shunts

I. Right-to-Left Shunts

A. Mnemonic: 5 T's

B. Tetralogy of fallot

C. Truncus arteriosus

D. Transposition

E. Tricuspid atresia

F. Total anomalous pulmonary venous return

G. Occurs when blood passes from the right to the left side of the heart without being oxygenated

1. V/Q mismatch

2. Hypoxemia

H. Present with early cyanosis

I. Urgent surgical treatment or maintenance of a PDA

II. Tetralogy of Fallot

A. Anterior and superior deviation of infundibular septum

B. "PROV"

1. Pulmonary infundibular stenosis

2. Right ventricular hypertrophy

3. Overriding aorta

4. Ventricular septal defects

C. Associated with fetal alcohol syndrome and 22q11 syndromes

D. Pulmonary stenosis → ↑ resistance near pulmonary artery → blood shunted from RV to systemic circulation

E. "Tet spells"

1. Hypercyanotic episodes

2. Mechanism is unclear but ultimately results in worsening of the shunt

3. Squatting improves symptoms (↑ SVR → ↑ pressure on the left side of the heart → reversal of shunt)

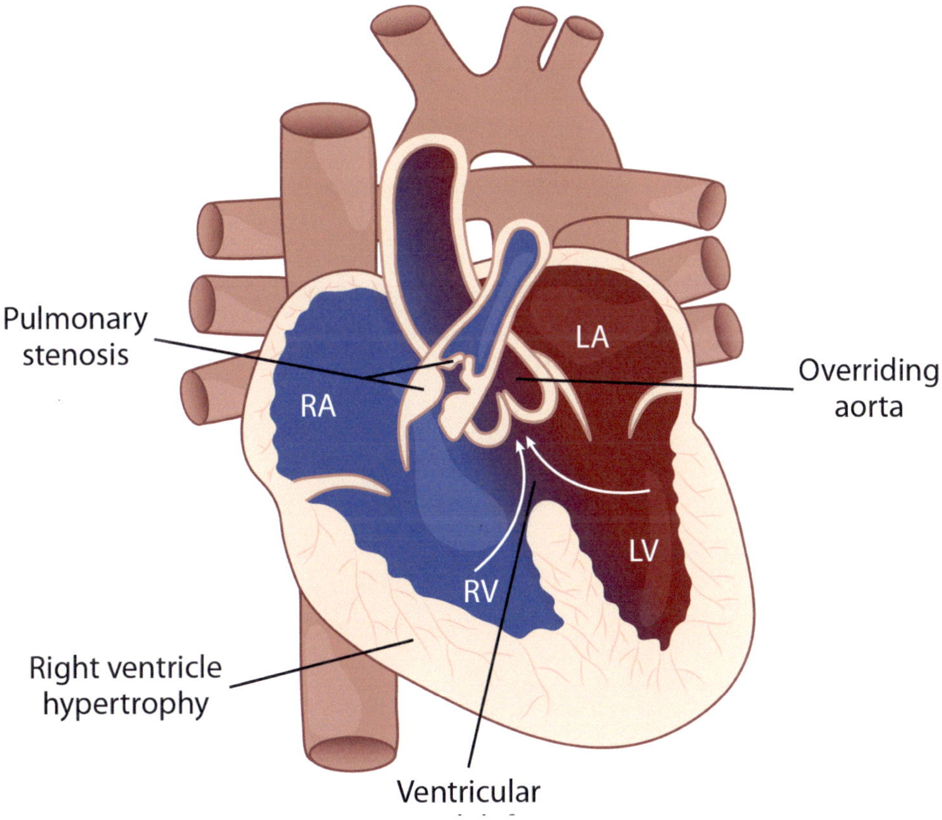

Figure 6.2.14- Tetralogy of Fallot

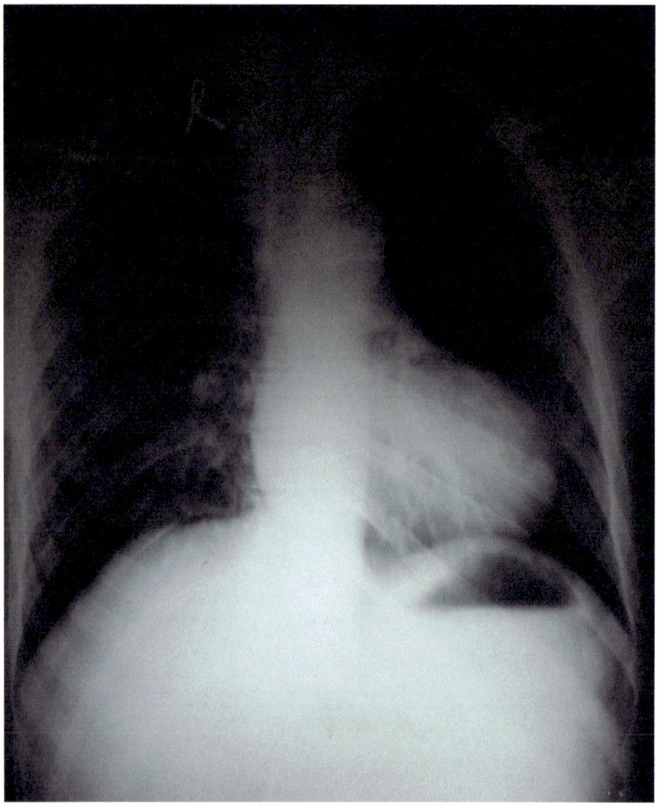

Figure 6.2.15 - Chest x-ray of Tetralogy of Fallot

III. Truncus Arteriosus

A. Aorticopulmonary septum fails to form

B. Commonly occurs with a VSD

C. Blood travels directly from the RV → aorta

D. Associated with 22q11 syndromes

IV. Transposition of Great Vessels

A. Failure of aorticopulmonary septum to spiral

1. Aorta arises from the right ventricle

2. Pulmonary artery arises from the left ventricle

B. Incompatible with life unless a shunt is present (eg, PDA, ASD, VSD)

C. Associated with infants of diabetic mothers

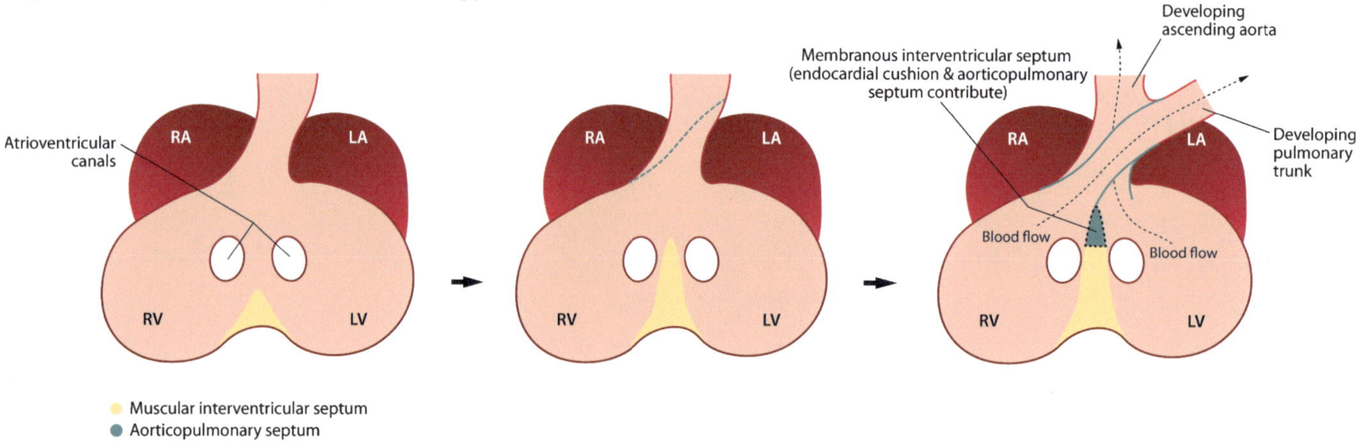

Figure 6.2.8 - Aorticopulmonary and muscular Interventricular septae

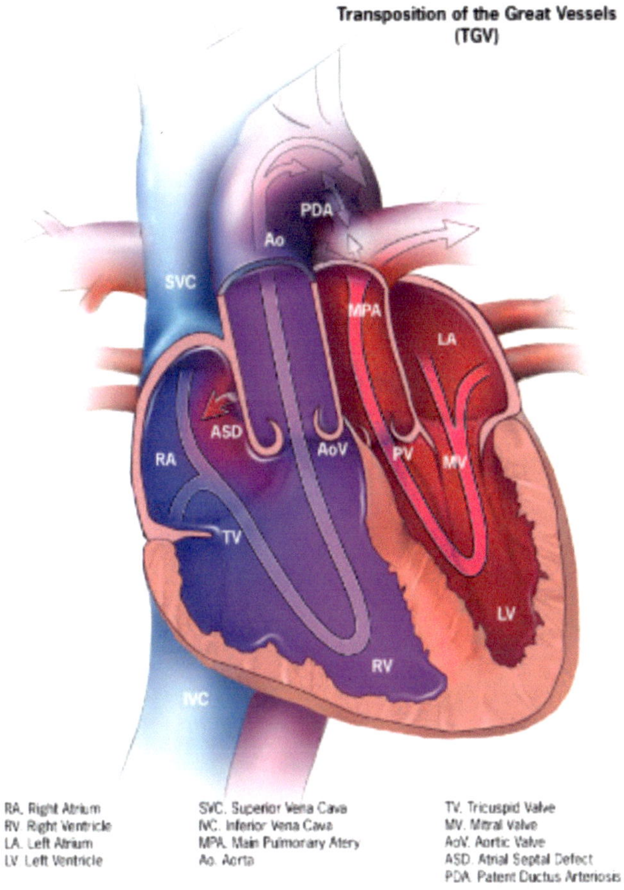

Photo Credit: Public Domain via CDC

Figure 6.2.16 - Transposition of the great vessels

V. Tricuspid Atresia

A. Congenital agenesis or absence of the tricuspid valve

1. No direct communication between right atrium and ventricle

B. Hypoplastic right ventricle

C. Incompatible with life unless a VSD and an ASD are present

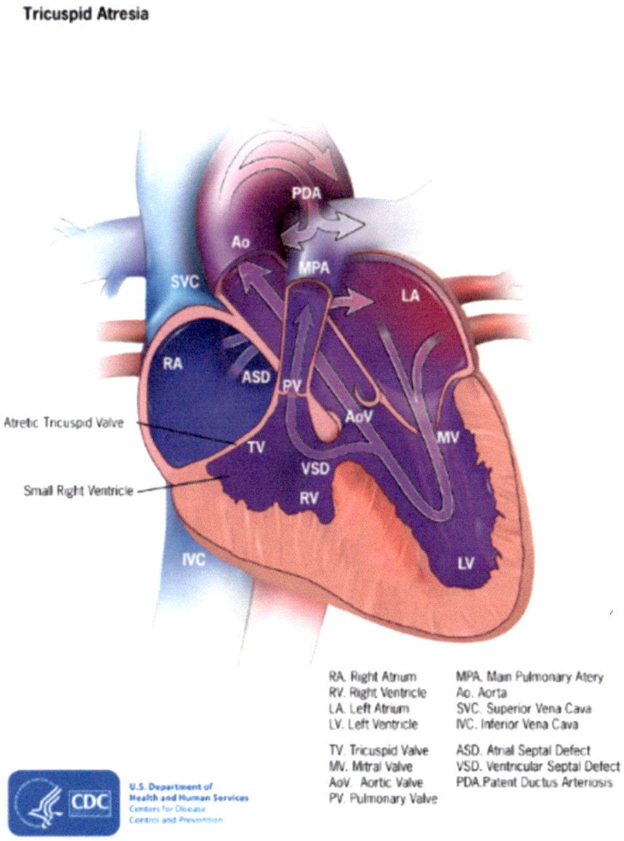

Photo Credit: Public Domain via CDC

Figure 6.2.17 - Tricuspid atresia

VI. Total Anomalous Pulmonary Venous Return

A. All four pulmonary veins fail to make a normal connection to the left atrium → blood drains into the systemic venous circulation

B. Left atrium fails to link with pulmonary venous plexus

C. Several variations depending on severity

D. Associated with an ASD

E. PDA may also be present

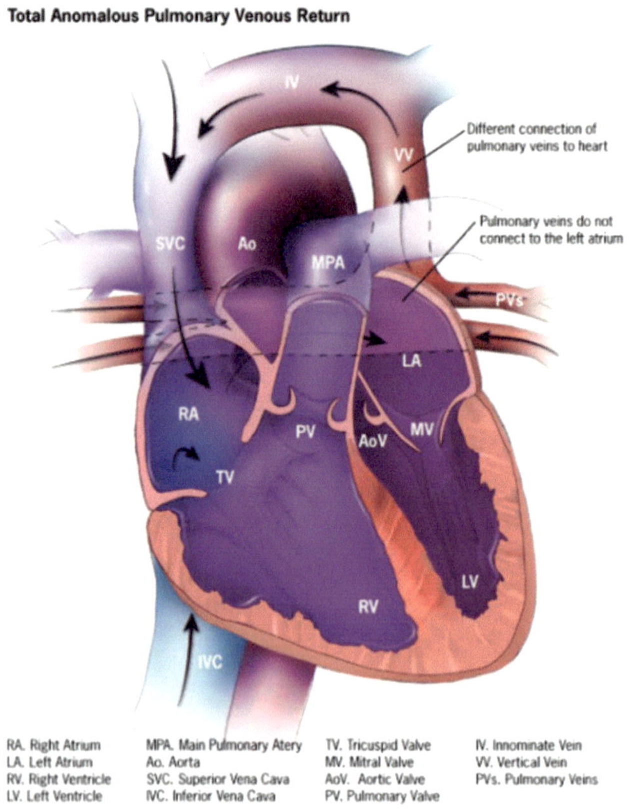

Photo Credit: Public Domain via CDC

Figure 6.2.18 - Total anomalous pulmonary venous return

VII. Ebstein Anomaly

A. Abnormalities of the tricuspid valve and right ventricle

1. Tricuspid valve is displaced towards apex
2. Right ventricle is "atrialized"

B. Associations:

1. Atrial septal defect
2. Tricuspid regurgitation
3. Accessory conduction pathways
4. Right-sided heart failure

C. Lithium exposure during pregnancy

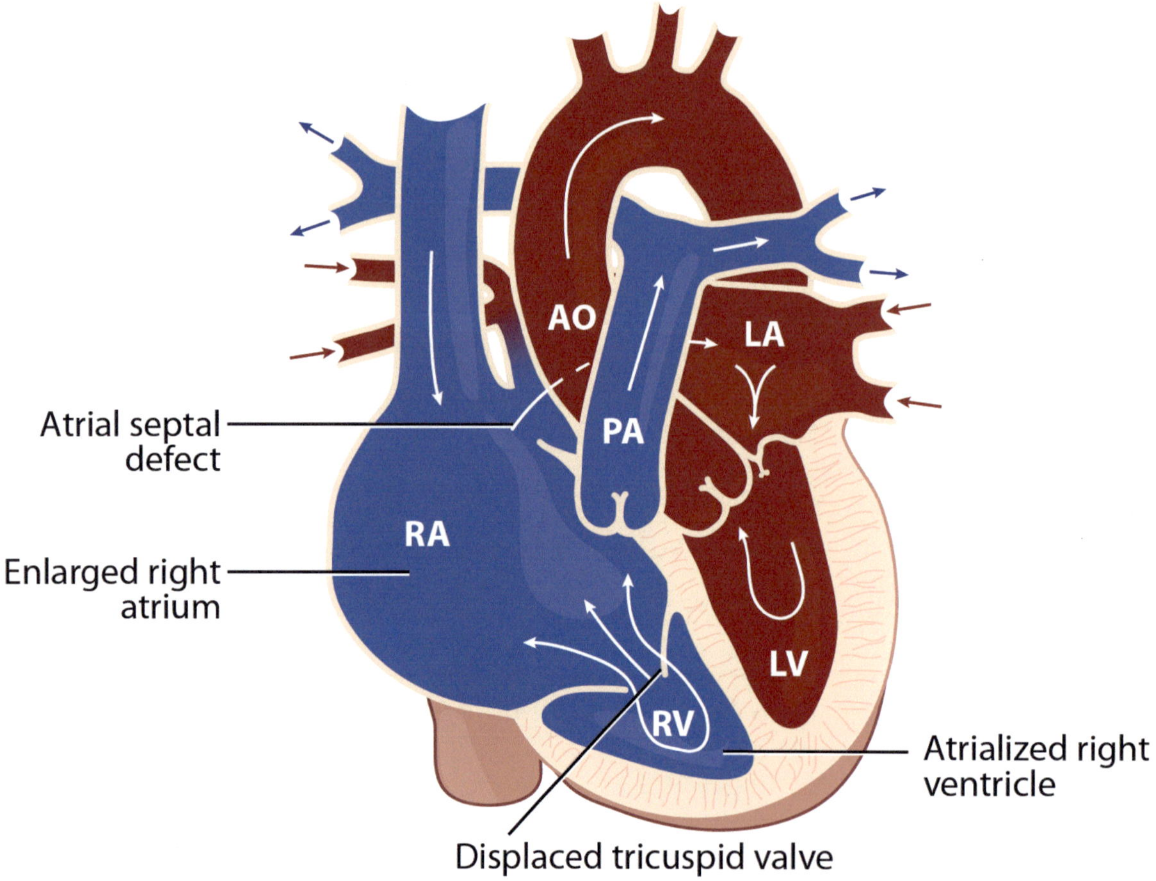

Figure 6.2.19 - Ebstein's anomaly

REVIEW QUESTIONS

1. A newborn male is found to have hypoxemia and cyanosis. A chest x-ray reveals a "boot-shaped" heart. The physician informs the parents that their child has a right-to-left cardiac shunt that will need to be surgically repaired. What are the four abnormal anatomical features associated with this patient's heart condition?

    - **The correct answer is pulmonary stenosis, right ventricular stenosis, overriding aorta, and ventricular septal defect.**
    - **Hypoxemia, cyanosis, and a boot-shaped heart are all highly suggestive of tetralogy of fallot.**
    - **This can be remembered with the mnemonic PROV.**
    - **P for pulmonary stenosis.**
    - **R for right ventricular hypertrophy.**
    - **O for overriding aorta**
    - **And V for ventricular septal defect.**

Section IV - Left-to-Right Shunts

I. Left-to-Right Shunt

A. Occurs when blood from the systemic arterial circulation mixes with systemic venous blood

1. Ventricular septal defect
2. Atrial septal defect
3. Patent ductus arteriosus

B. Newborns are acyanotic (cyanosis may present later)

C. Eisenmenger syndrome is a potential complication

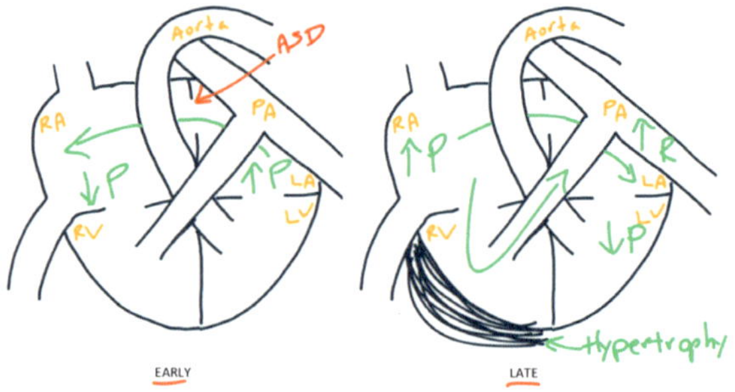

II. Eisenmenger Syndrome

A. Chronic left-to-right shunt → ↑ pulmonary blood flow → ↑ pulmonary vascular resistance → ↑ RV pressure / RV hypertrophy → reversal of shunt

B. Clinical presentation:

1. Central cyanosis
2. Digital clubbing
3. Polycythemia

C. Time course of reversal varies

III. Ventricular Septal Defect

A. Second most common congenital heart defect (bicuspid aortic valve most common)

B. Often asymptomatic at birth and close spontaneously

C. Large VSDs → Eisenmenger syndrome and heart failure

D. Holosystolic murmur

E. ↑ O_2 saturation on the right side of the heart

F. Infants of diabetic mother, fetal alcohol syndrome, Down syndrome

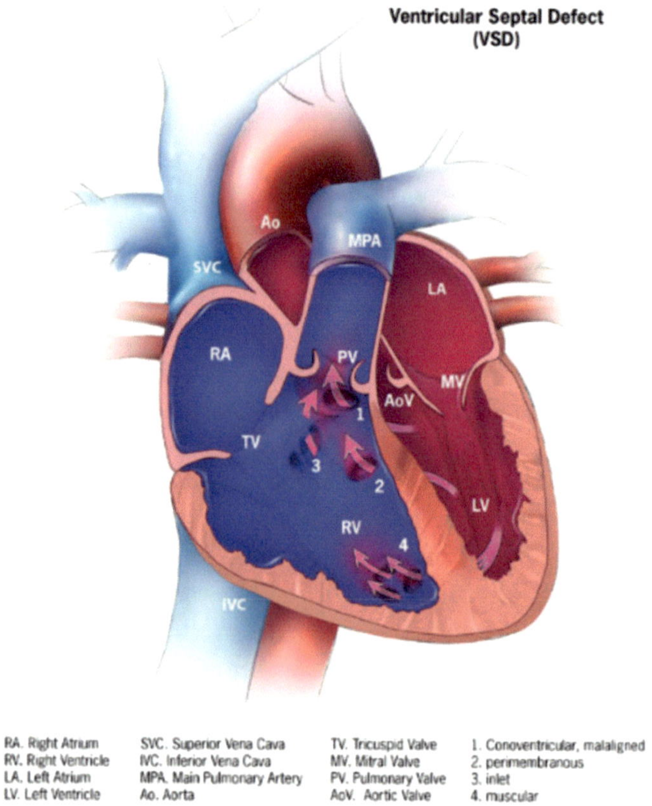

Photo Credit: Public Domain via CDC

Figure 6.2.20 - Ventricular septal defect

IV. Atrial Septal Defect

A. 10-15 percent of congenital heart disease

B. Classified by anatomic location

C. Primum

1. Septum primum doesn't fuse with the endocardial cushion
2. Occurs with other anomalies (eg, AV canal defects, VSDs)

D. Secundum

1. Arrested growth of the second septum → opening in the fossa ovalis
2. More common
3. Isolated finding

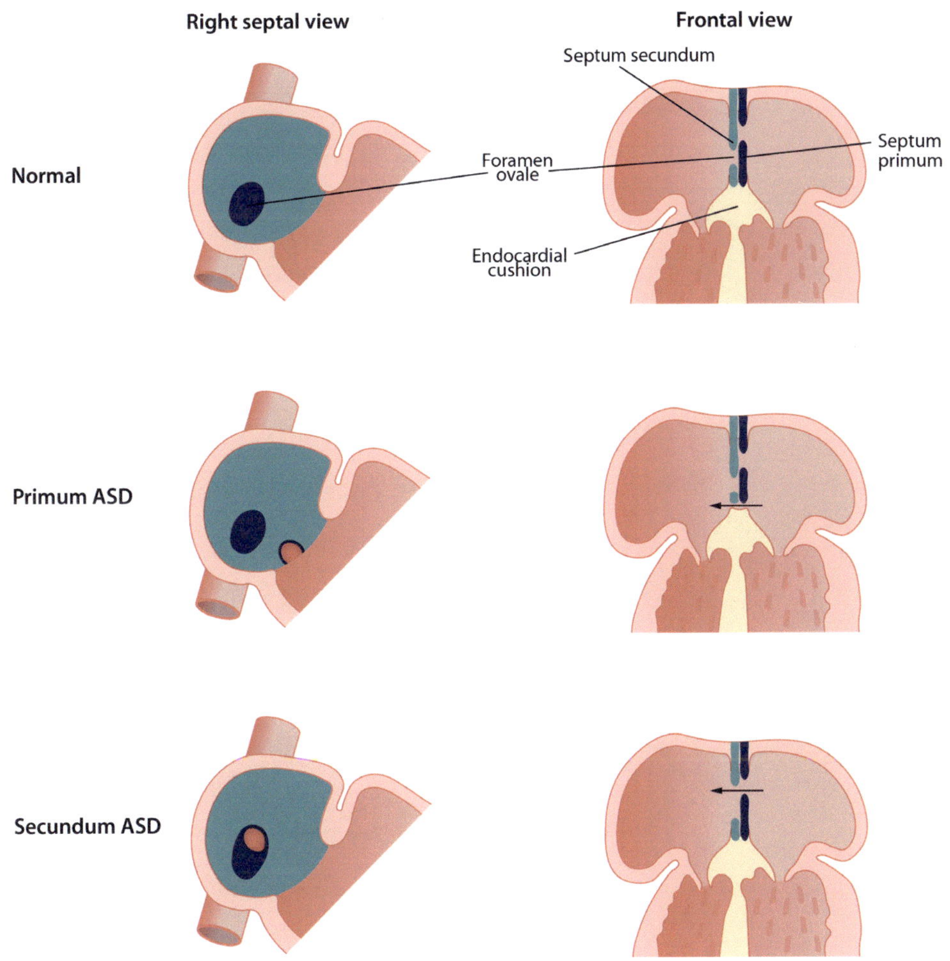

Figure 6.2.21 - Interatrial septum formation and defects

E. Delayed closure of the pulmonic valve
F. Systolic ejection murmur
G. Fixed split of S2
H. Signs of heart failure
I. Venous emboli → arterial emboli
J. ↑ O_2 saturation on the right side of the heart
K. Associated with fetal alcohol syndrome and Down syndrome

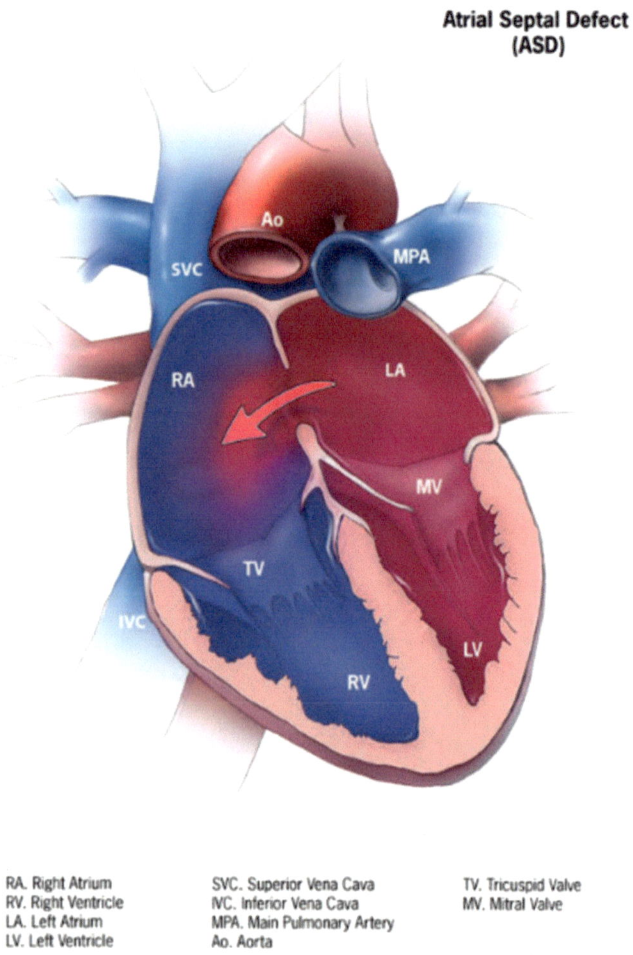

Photo Credit: Public Domain via CDC

Figure 6.2.22 - Atrial septal defect

V. Patent Ductus Arteriosus

A. Ductus arteriosus is derived from left sixth aortic arch

B. Fetal vascular connection between main pulmonary artery and aorta

C. Patency maintained by low arterial oxygen and prostaglandin E2

D. Constricts and obliterates after birth

E. PDA persists up to or beyond 6 weeks after birth

F. Females >>> males

G. Congenital rubella

H. Prematurity

I. High altitude

J. Clinical presentation depends on size and length of PDA:

1. Generally asymptomatic
2. “Machine-like” murmur
3. Right and left ventricular hypertrophy
4. Cyanosis of the lower limbs
5. Widened pulse pressure

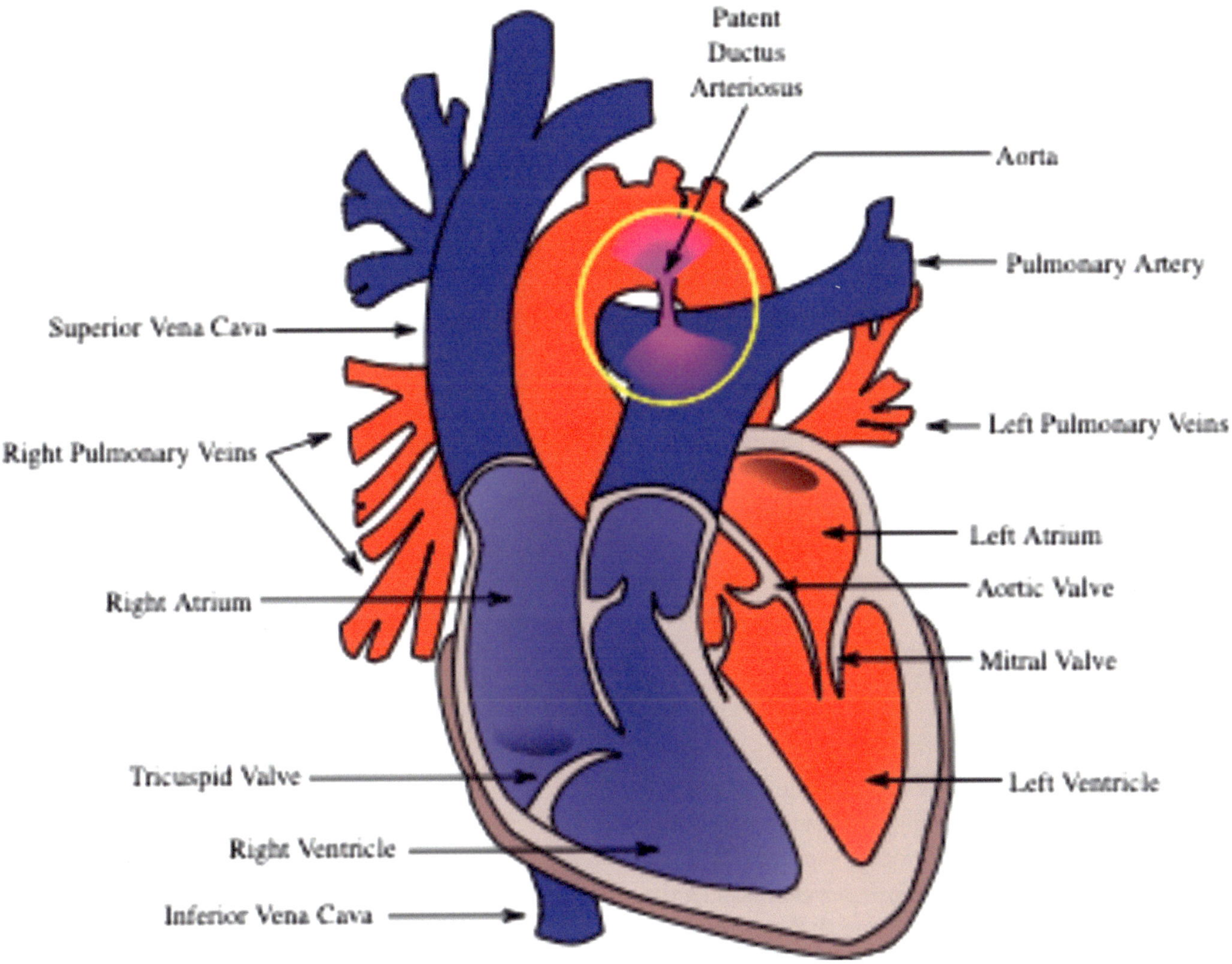

Photo Credit: BrownCow. [Public domain]

Figure 6.2.23 - Patent ductus arteriosus

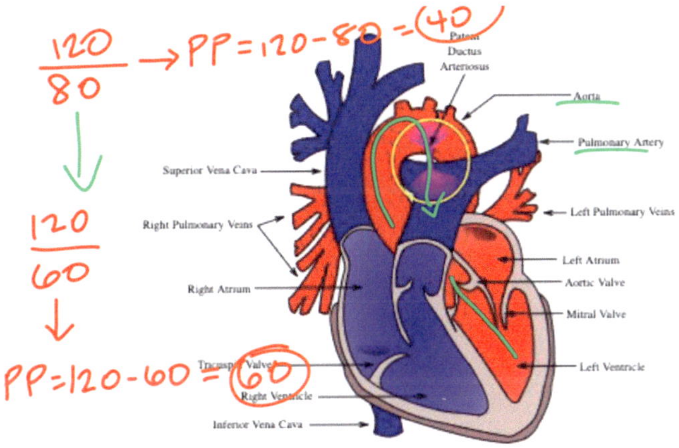

REVIEW QUESTIONS ?

1. A 21-year-old male presents to the emergency department due to left-sided weakness and slurred speech after a long flight. Auscultation of the left sternal border reveals a systolic ejection murmur. An echocardiogram reveals that an area of tissue is missing at the opening of the fossa ovalis. What type of septal defect is most likely present in this individual?

- **Secundum atrial septal defect.**
- **This patient had left-sided weakness and slurred speech after a long flight which is highly suggestive of a stroke.**
- **The long flight idea is important because it's alluding to the idea that the patient was exposed to hemostasis which then resulted in a deep venous thrombosis.**
- **Hemostasis → DVT → bypass lungs → stroke.**
- **The physical examination of the heart that revealed a systolic ejection murmur along with the echocardiogram confirms that this patient has an interatrial septal defect.**
- **It's not a patent foramen ovale because the echocardiogram revealed that an area of tissue is missing.**
- **In a PFO the tissue is present, the interatrial septum just hasn't fully closed after birth.**
- **The location of the defect is at the opening of the fossa ovalis which means that this patient has a secundum atrial septal defect.**

PULMONOLOGY

Section I - Respiratory Embryology

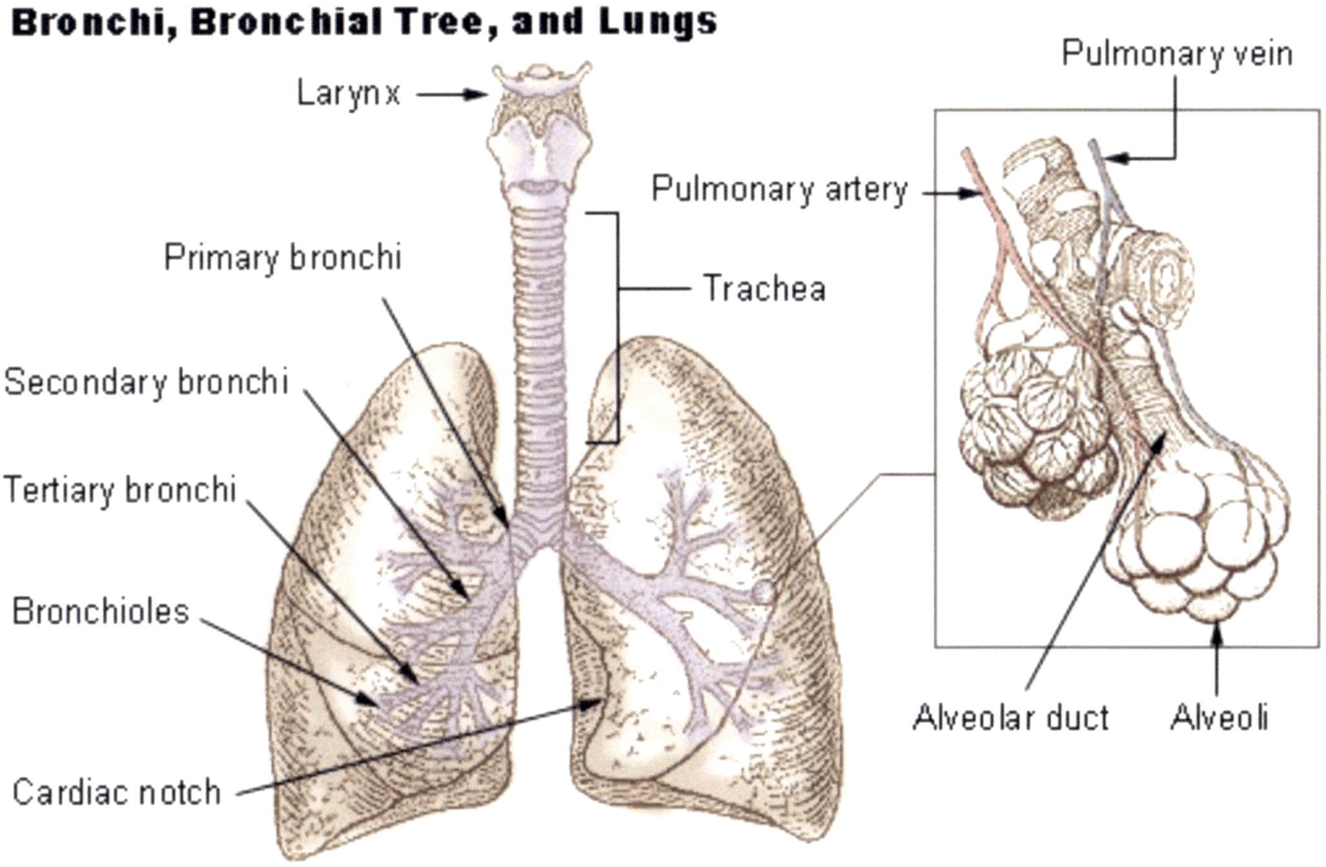

Photo Credit: [Public Domain]

Figure 6.3.1 - Bronchi, bronchial tree, and lungs

I. Five Stages of Lung Development

   A. Five stages

      1. Embryonic
      2. Pseudoglandular
      3. Canalicular
      4. Saccular
      5. Alveolar

   B. Mnemonic: "Every Pulmonologist Can See Alveoli"

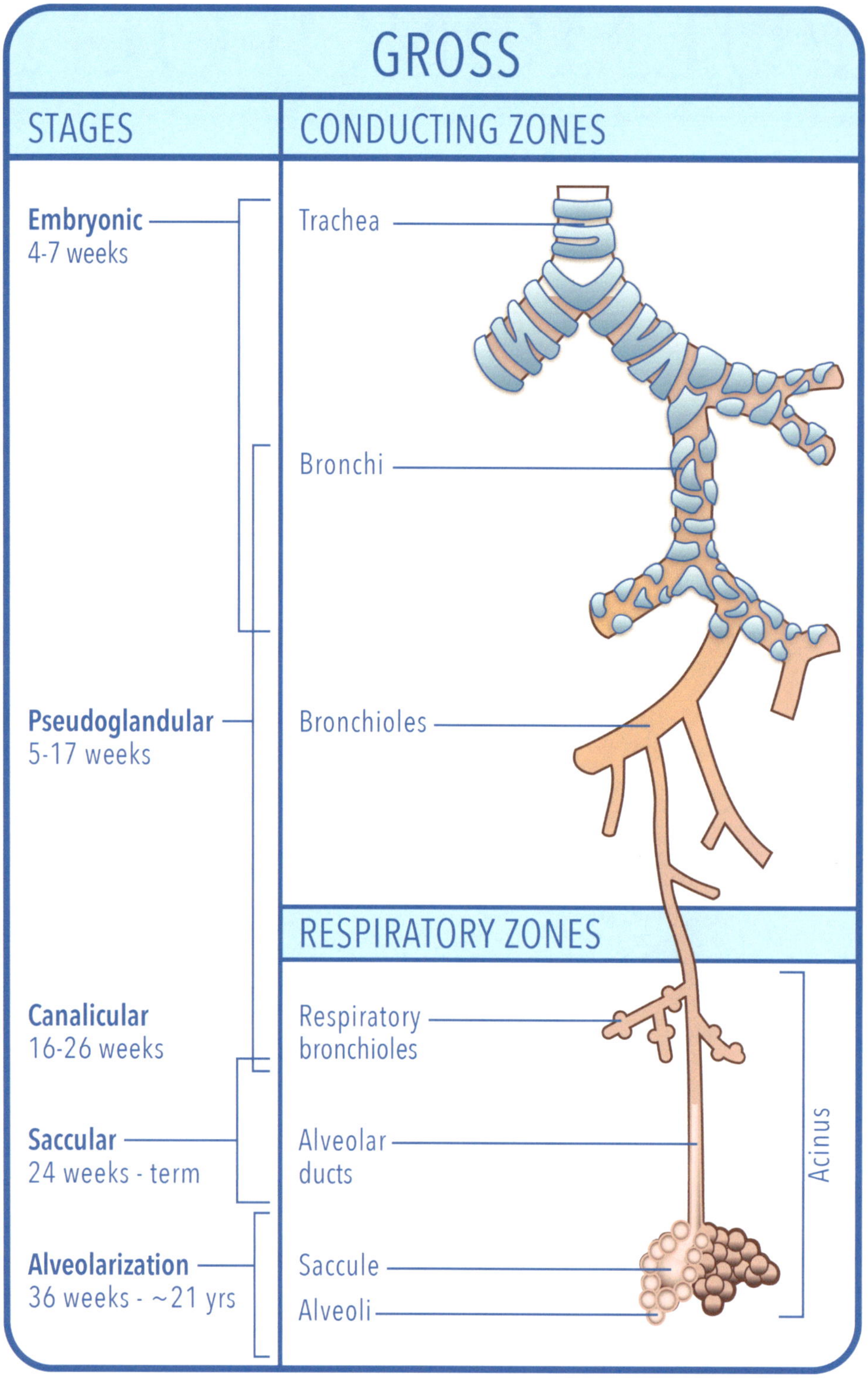

Figure 6.3.2 - Anatomy of the respiratory tree

II. Embryonic Stage (weeks 4-7)

A. Respiratory diverticulum (foregut) → trachea develops → esophagus and trachea separate

B. Errors in this stage lead to tracheoesophageal fistula (TEF) and/or esophageal atresia (EA)

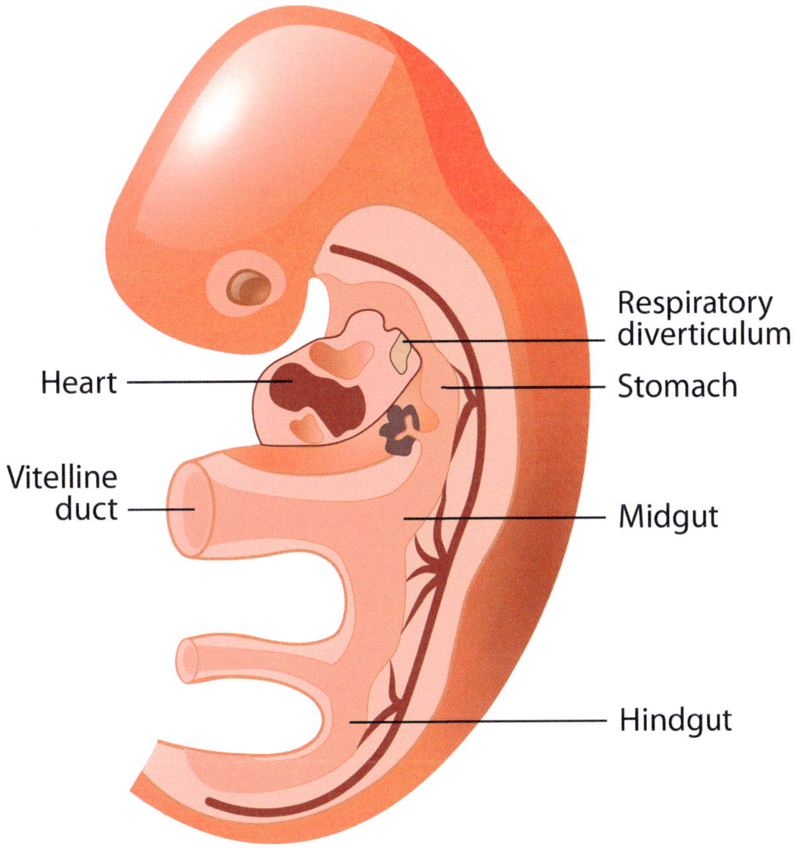

Figure 6.3.3 - Lateral view of respiratory diverticulum

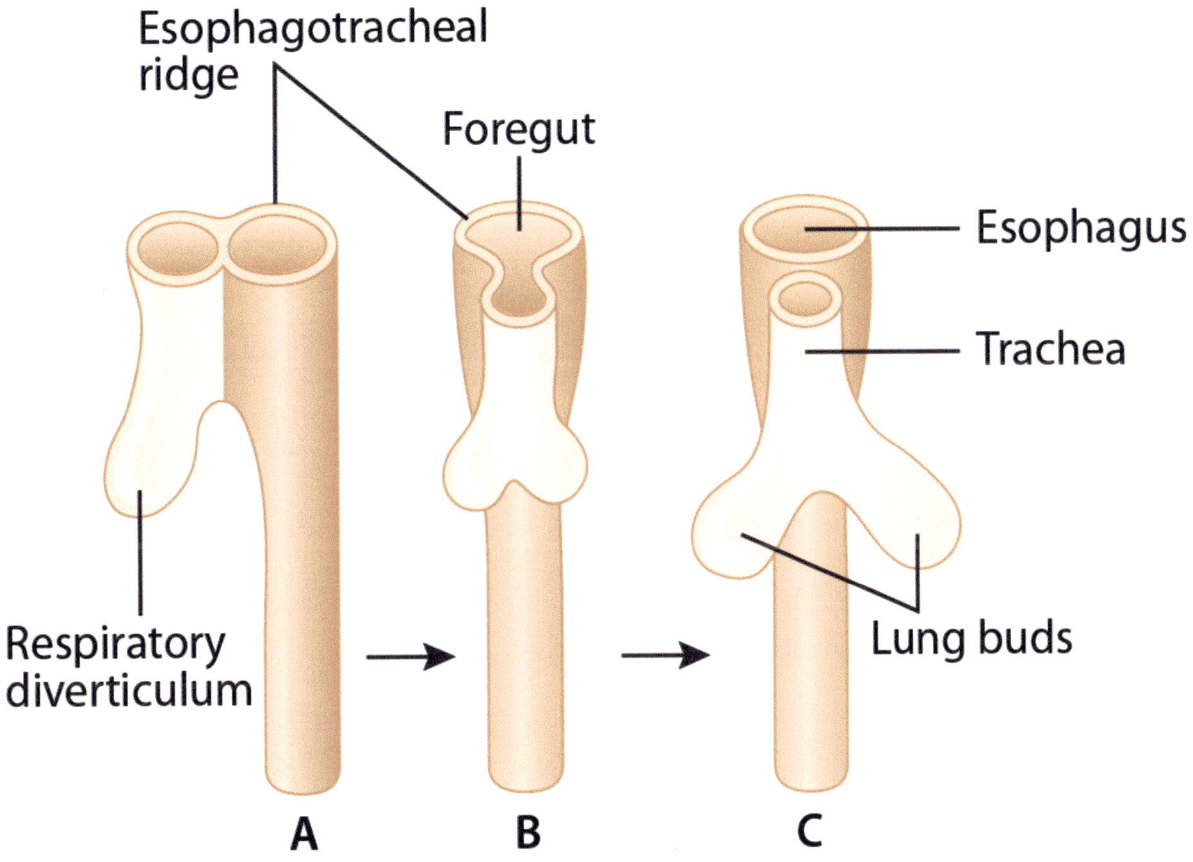

Figure 6.3.4 - Development of lung buds from the foregut

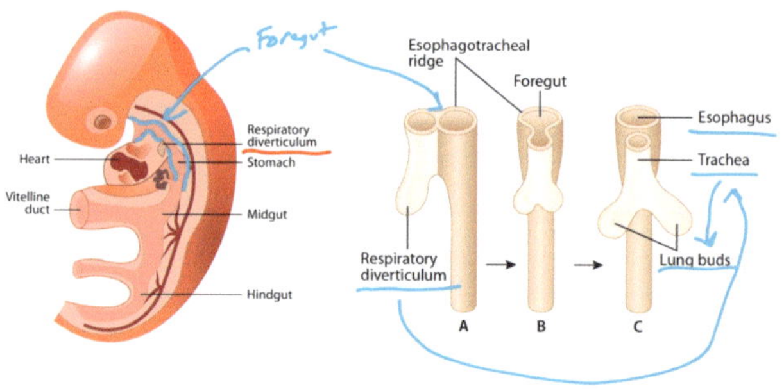

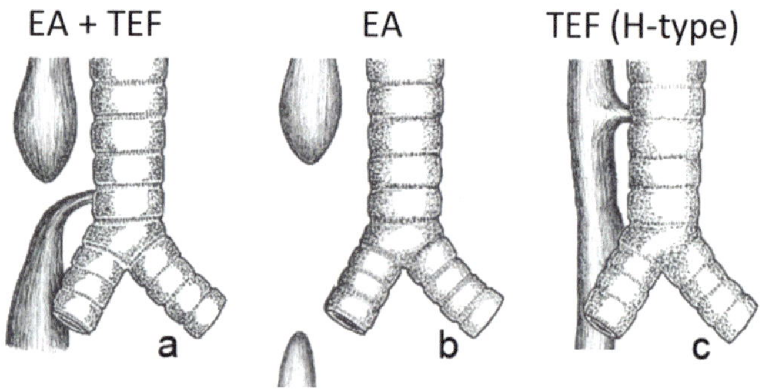

Photo Credit: Lewis Spitz. Oesophageal atresia. Orphanet Journal of Rare Diseases. 2, 24. 2007.

Figure 6.3.5 - Depiction of esophageal atresia and tracheoesophageal fistula

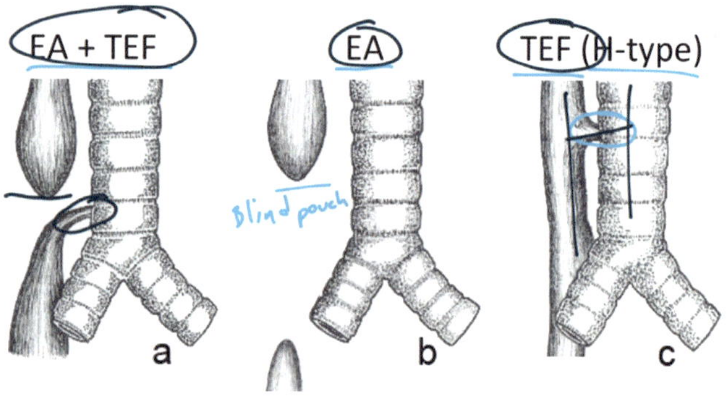

III. Presentation of Esophageal Atresia (EA) and Tracheoesophageal Fistula (TEF)

   A. Esophageal atresia

      1. Drooling, choking, vomiting on first feed

      2. Polyhydramnios

   B. Tracheoesophageal fistula

      1. Gastric distension

      2. Aspiration pneumonia

IV. Diagnosis and Treatment of EA, EA + TEF, and pure TEF (H-type)

   A. EA or EA + TEF

      1. Diagnosis: Nasogastric tube fails to enter stomach

      2. Treatment: Surgery

   B. Pure TEF (H-type)

      1. Diagnosis: Visualize using fluoroscopy (x-ray with dye)

      2. Treatment: Surgery

V. Bronchogenic Cysts

   A. Abnormal budding of the foregut (mediastinum)

   B. Typically asymptomatic

   C. Respiratory epithelium w/ cartilage

   D. Fluid filled (air filled if infected)

      1. Poorly draining

VI. Pseudoglandular Stage (weeks 5-17)

   A. Respiration still not possible (incompatible with life)

   B. Terminal bronchioles

   C. Capillary network

   D. Fetal respiration

      1. Aspiration of small amounts of amniotic fluid → stimulates lung growth and development

VII. Pulmonary Hypoplasia

   A. Poor development of bronchopulmonary tree

      1. Potter's sequence

      2. Diaphragmatic hernia

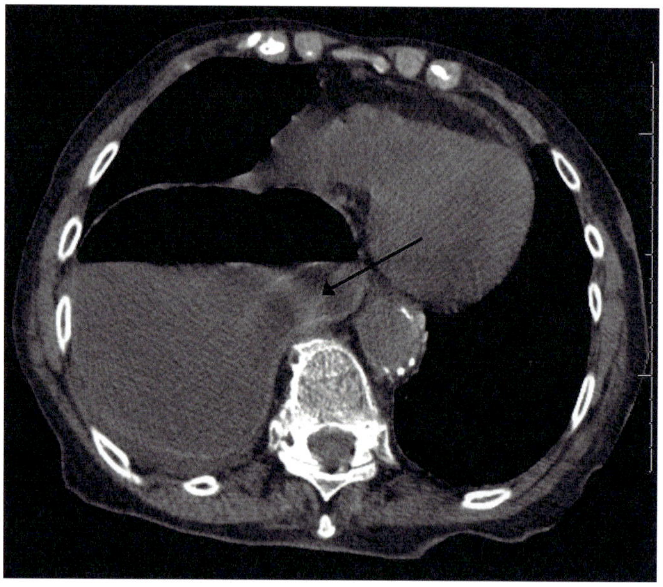

Photo Credit: James Heilman, MD [CC BY-SA 3.0 (https://creativecommons.org/licenses/by-sa/3.0)]

Figure 6.3.6 - Axial MRI of diaphragmatic hernia

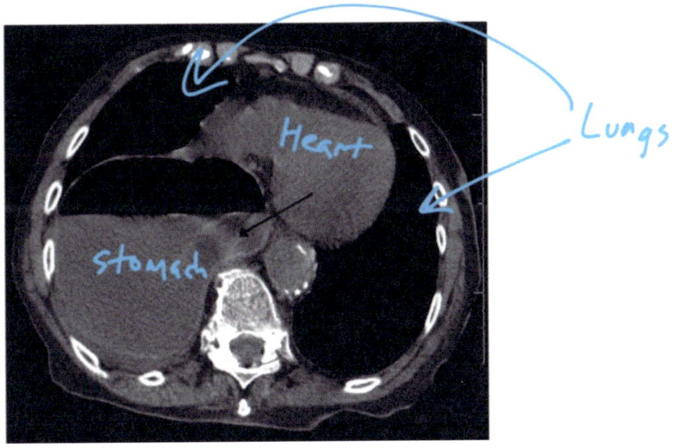

VIII. Canalicular Stage (weeks 16-25)

A. Formation of:

1. Respiratory bronchioles
2. Alveolar ducts
3. Stronger capillary network
4. Type II pneumocytes (20 weeks)

B. Respiration possible

IX. Saccular Stage (weeks 26-36, birth)

A. Formation of:

1. Terminal sacs with primary septae

X. Alveolar Stage (weeks 36-8 years)

A. Formation of:

1. Adult alveoli - secondary septae
2. From ~35 million to 350 million
3. Disruption can cause bronchopulmonary dysplasia

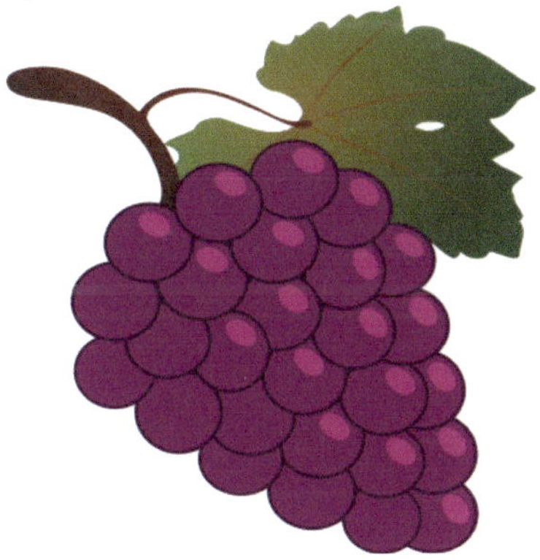

Photo Credit: Jean Victor Balin [CC0]

REVIEW QUESTIONS ?

1. A newborn baby is born with flattened facies and clubfeet. On further inspection it is found that the baby has pulmonary hypoplasia. Which disturbance in lung development would most likely lead to the symptoms described?

A. Abnormal budding of the foregut
B. Diaphragmatic hernia
C. Polyhydramnios
D. Failure of trachea to separate from foregut
E. Renal agenesis

- **Answer: E, renal agenesis**
- **Flattened facies, clubfeet, and pulmonary hypoplasia are findings consistent with Potter syndrome. The only option listed that can result in oligohydramnios and Potter syndrome is renal agenesis**
- **A is incorrect because abnormal budding of the foregut causes bronchogenic cysts**
- **B is incorrect because diaphragmatic hernia causes pulmonary hypoplasia but none of the other symptoms**
- **Polyhydramnios is too much amniotic fluid which is the opposite of oligohydramnios.**
- **D is incorrect because failure of the trachea to separate from the foregut causes esophageal atresia with or without tracheal-esophageal fistula**

NEPHROLOGY

Section I - Normal Renal Development

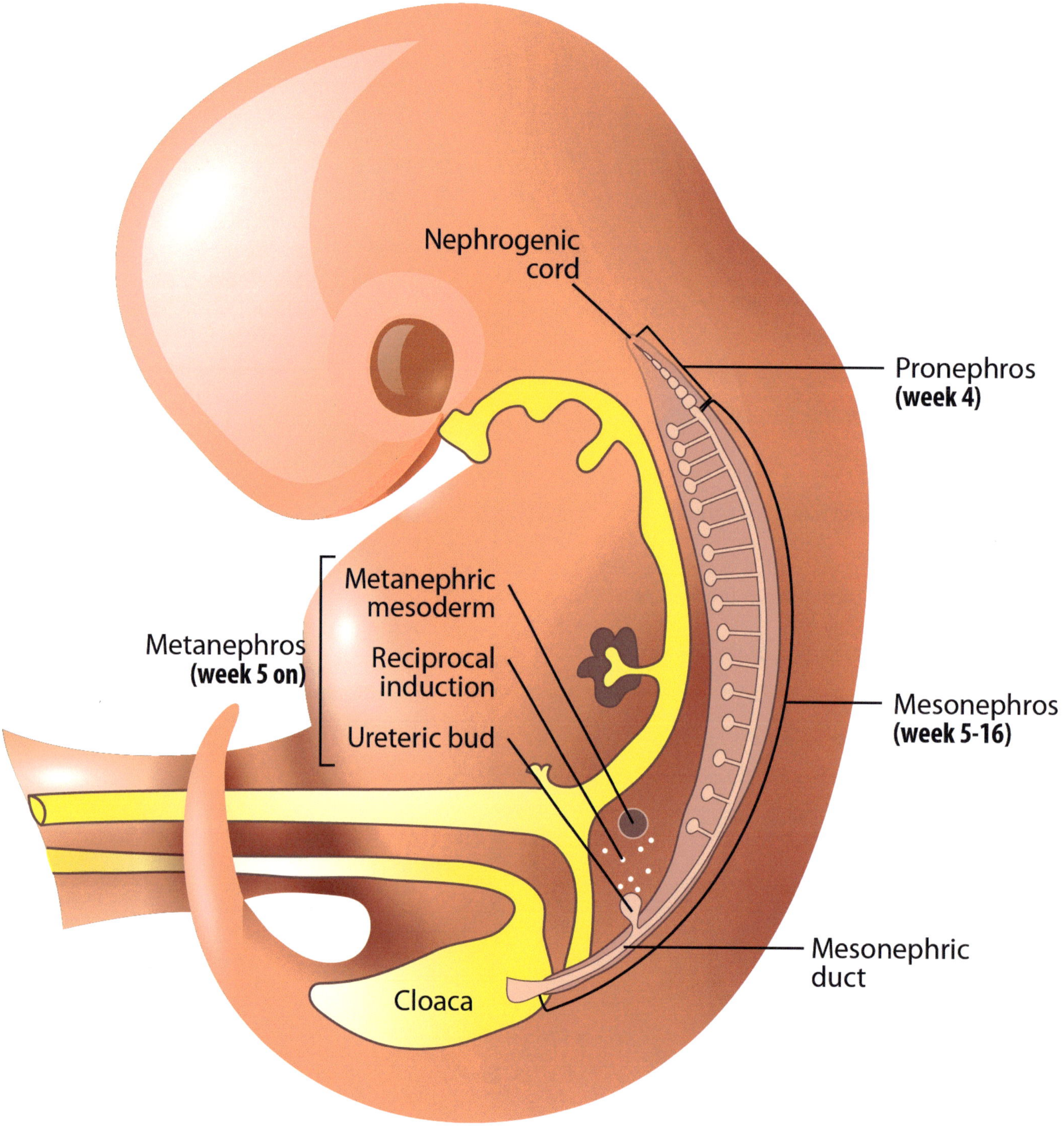

Figure 6.4.1 - Fetal development of urinary system

Stage	Timing	Muscles
Pronephros	• Develops and degenerates during week 4	• Does not excrete filtered material (non-functional)
Mesonephros	• Develops around week 5 • Functions as a temporary kidney • Regresses by week 16	• Develops mesonephric duct (early urine filtration drain) → gives rise to the ureteric bud (see metanephros below) • Mesonephric duct degenerates and forms the Wolffian duct → forms internal male genitalia (except prostate)

Metanephros	• Starts forming in week 5
	• Fully canalized and functional by week 10
		• The mesonephric duct and the metanephric mesoderm (blastema) interact (reciprocal induction)
		  • Mesonephric duct → ureteric bud (metanephrogenic diverticulum) → collecting system (collecting duct through ureter)
		  • Metanephric mesoderm (blastema) → filtration system (glomerulus through DCT)
		• Mature kidney migrates from the pelvis to the lumbar region

Table 6.4.1 - Development of the urinary system in utero

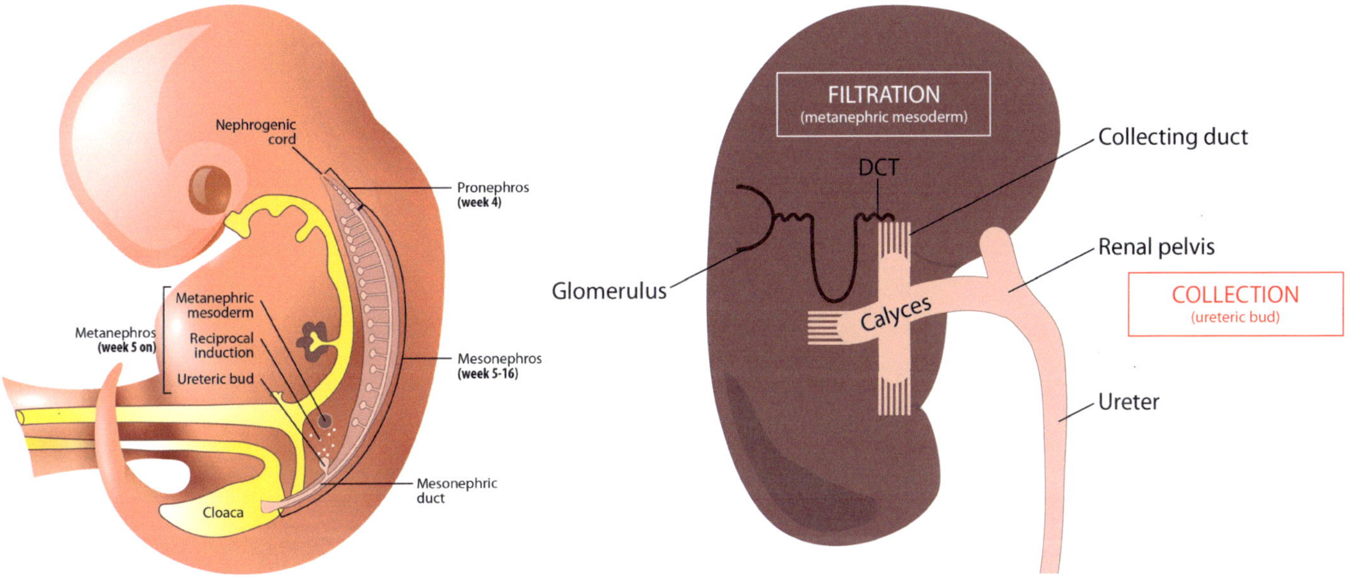

Figure 6.4.2 - Development of filtration and collections systems from fetus to adult

I. Urine through Pregnancy

A. First trimester

1. Mesonephric duct → cloaca → allantois/ urachus → umbilical cord

B. Second and third trimester

1. Kidney → ureter → bladder → urethra → amniotic fluid

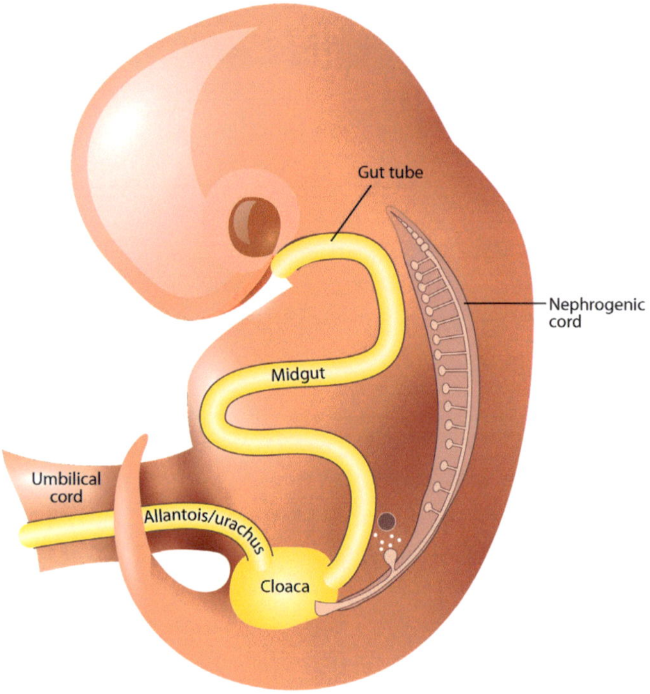

Figure 6.2.11 - Urinary excretion in 1st trimester

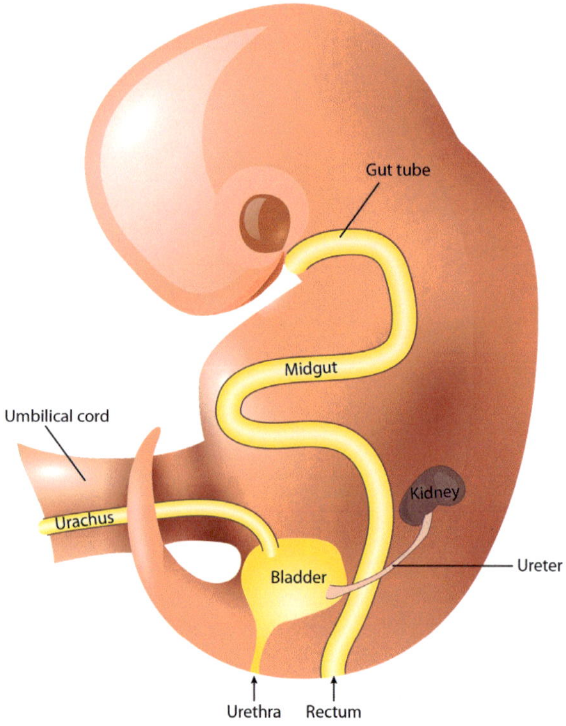

Figure 6.2.11- Urinary excretion in 2nd and 3rd trimesters

II. Urachus

A. Connects bladder to umbilicus

B. Normally obliterates during the second trimester and becomes the median umbilical ligament in adults

C. Failure to obliterate can lead to various pathologies, all of which increase risk of infection and adenocarcinoma of the bladder

1. Patent urachus → urine from umbilicus

2. Urachal cyst → painful mass

3. Vesicourachal diverticulum → bladder outpouching

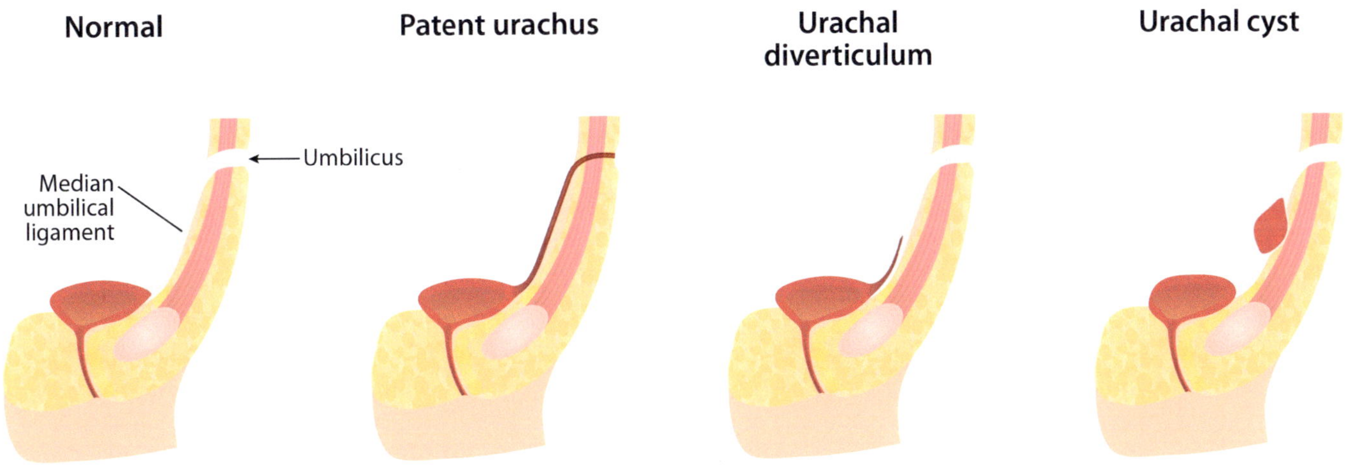

Figure 6.4.3 - Urachal pathologies

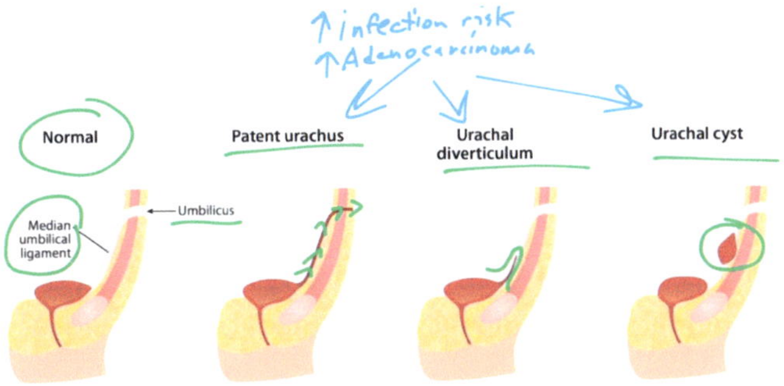

REVIEW QUESTIONS

1. A researcher is studying the transporters on the proximal convoluted tubule (PCT) of the nephron. What embryological structure gave rise to the PCT?

    - **Answer: The metanephric mesoderm**
    - **The filtration system comes from metanephric mesoderm, including everything from the glomerulus to the distal convoluted tubule, which includes the proximal convoluted tubule**
    - **Conversely, the collection system is derived from the ureteric bud, which branched off the mesonephric duct**

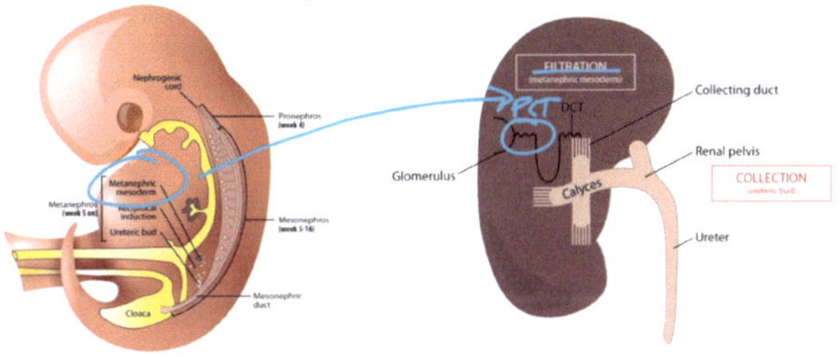

Section II - Pathology of Renal Development

Pathology	Pathophysiology	Clinical Outcome
Potter syndrome	- Failure to excrete urine into the amniotic fluid → oligohydramnios - Insufficient urine excretion can be caused by many issues including placental insufficiency, renal agenesis, MCDK, ARPKD, posterior urethral valves	- Oligohydramnios causes multiple issues: - ↓ protective cushioning → fetal compression → twisted face, and skin and extremity defects - ↓ fluid inhaled into lungs → lungs compressed & unable to fully develop → pulmonary hypoplasia
Renal agenesis	- Ureteric bud fails to develop → metanephros development does not occur (metanephric mesoderm and ureteric bud require reciprocal induction to form a kidney)	- Bilateral pathology → insufficient urine excretion → oligohydramnios and Potter syndrome - Unilateral pathology → hyperfiltration of the developed kidney → renal hypertrophy and risk of renal failure
Multicystic dysplastic kidney (MCDK)	- Ureteric bud and metanephric mesoderm interact abnormally → metanephric mesoderm fails to differentiate → nonfunctional kidney and formation of cysts and cartilage → ↓ urine excretion	
Autosomal recessive polycystic kidney disease (ARPKD)	- Autosomal recessive cystic dilation of renal collecting ducts in both kidneys → bilateral kidney enlargement → renal failure → ↓ urine excretion	- Potter syndrome
Posterior urethral valve	- Occurs in males - Membranous remnant of the male urethral valve - Located at the bladder-urethral junction → obstruction → enlarged, hypertrophied bladder → ↓ urine excretion - High bladder pressure → vesicoureteral reflux → hydronephrosis	- Potter syndrome - Recurrent UTIs
Ureteropelvic junction obstruction	- Junction near the renal pelvis and ureter fail to canalize → urine cannot pass the ureteropelvic junction → urine builds up in kidney → hydronephrosis - Often occurs alongside vesicoureteral reflux	- Bilateral pathology → recurrent UTIs and Potter syndrome - Unilateral pathology (most common) → recurrent UTIs
Duplex collecting systems	- Unilateral bifurcation of the ureteric bud before contacting the metanephric mesenchyme → duplicated (bifid) ureter - The duplicated (ectopic) ureter is narrow → obstruction → hydronephrosis - The narrow ureter may attach directly to the bladder → vesicoureteral reflux	- Recurrent UTIs
Horseshoe kidney	- Associated with Turner syndrome and trisomies 13, 18, and 21 - Inferior poles of both kidneys fuse together → horseshoe-shaped kidney → cannot ascend past inferior mesenteric artery → kidneys remain in lower abdomen → obstruction and/or vesicoureteral reflux → hydronephrosis	- Recurrent UTIs - Renal stones

Table 6.4.2 - Pathology of Renal Development

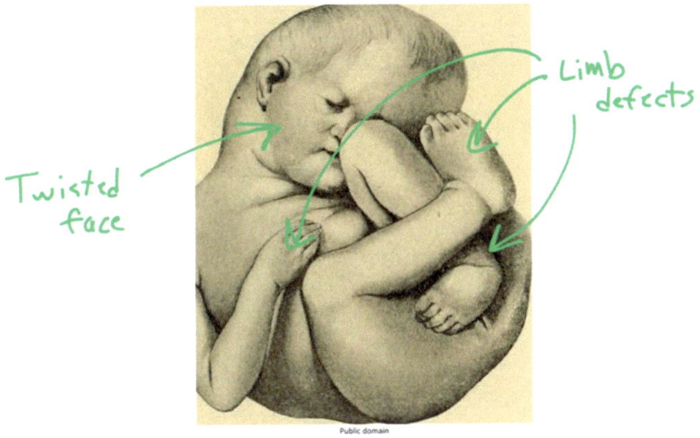

Figure 4.4

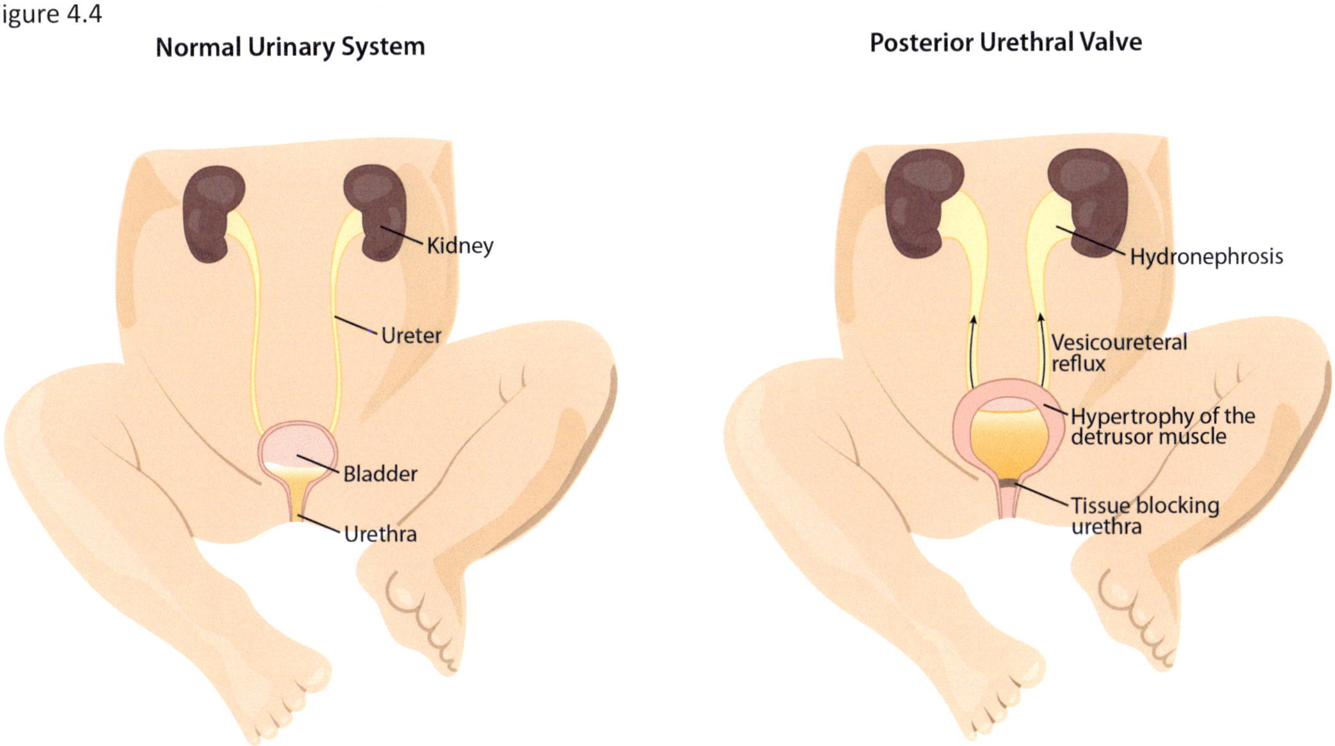

Figure 6.4.5 - Posterior urethral valve

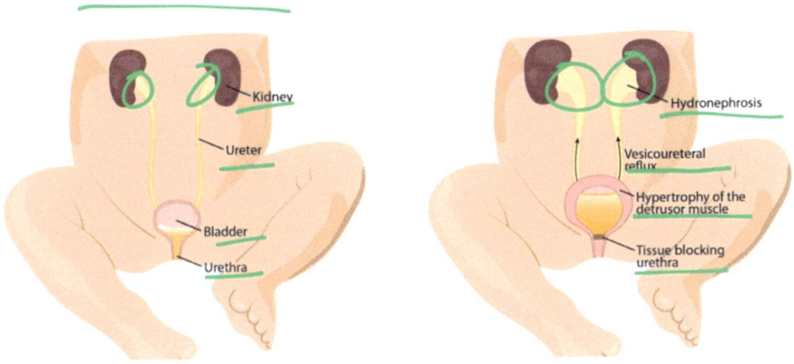

1. Ureteropelvic Junction Obstruction

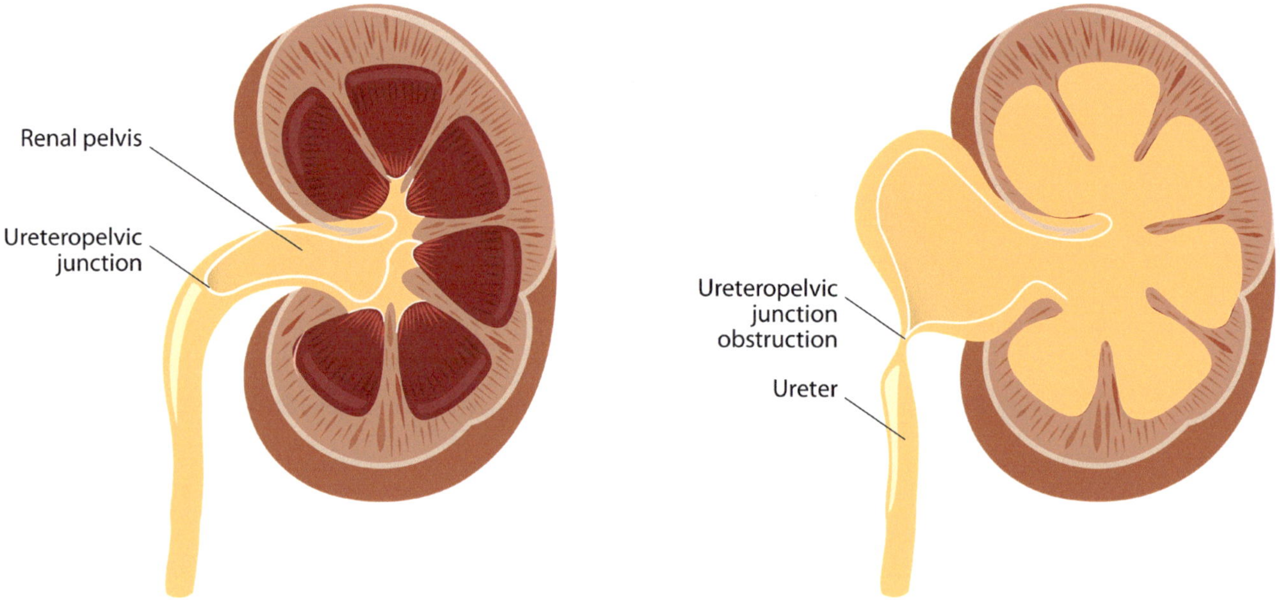

Figure 6.4.6 - Ureteropelvic junction obstruction

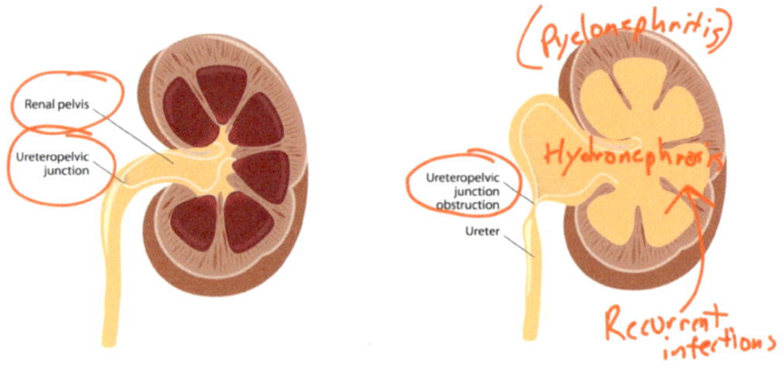

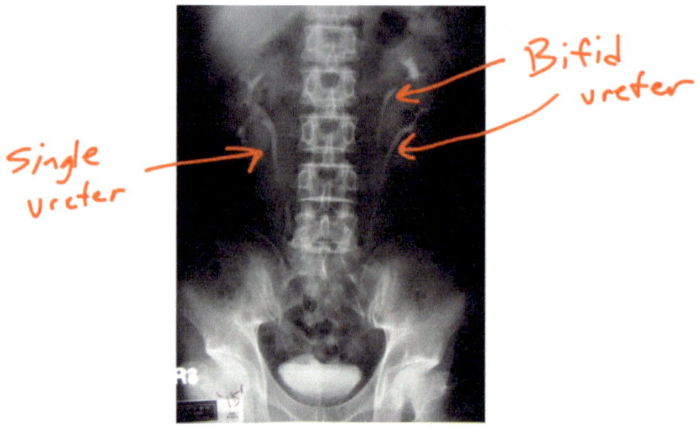

Photo Credit: No machine-readable author provided. Morning2k assumed (based on copyright claims).

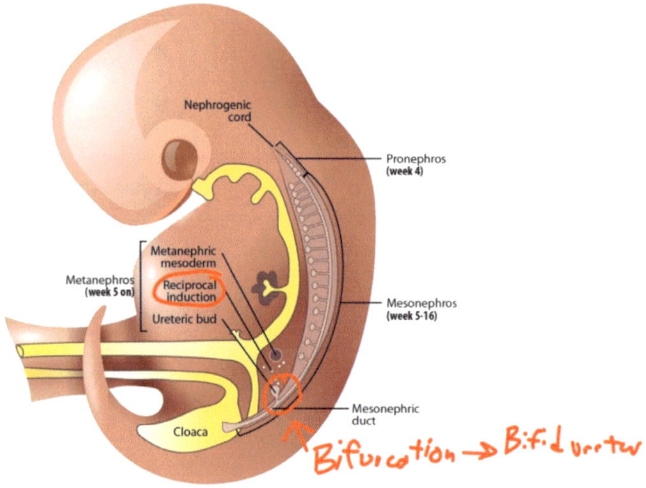

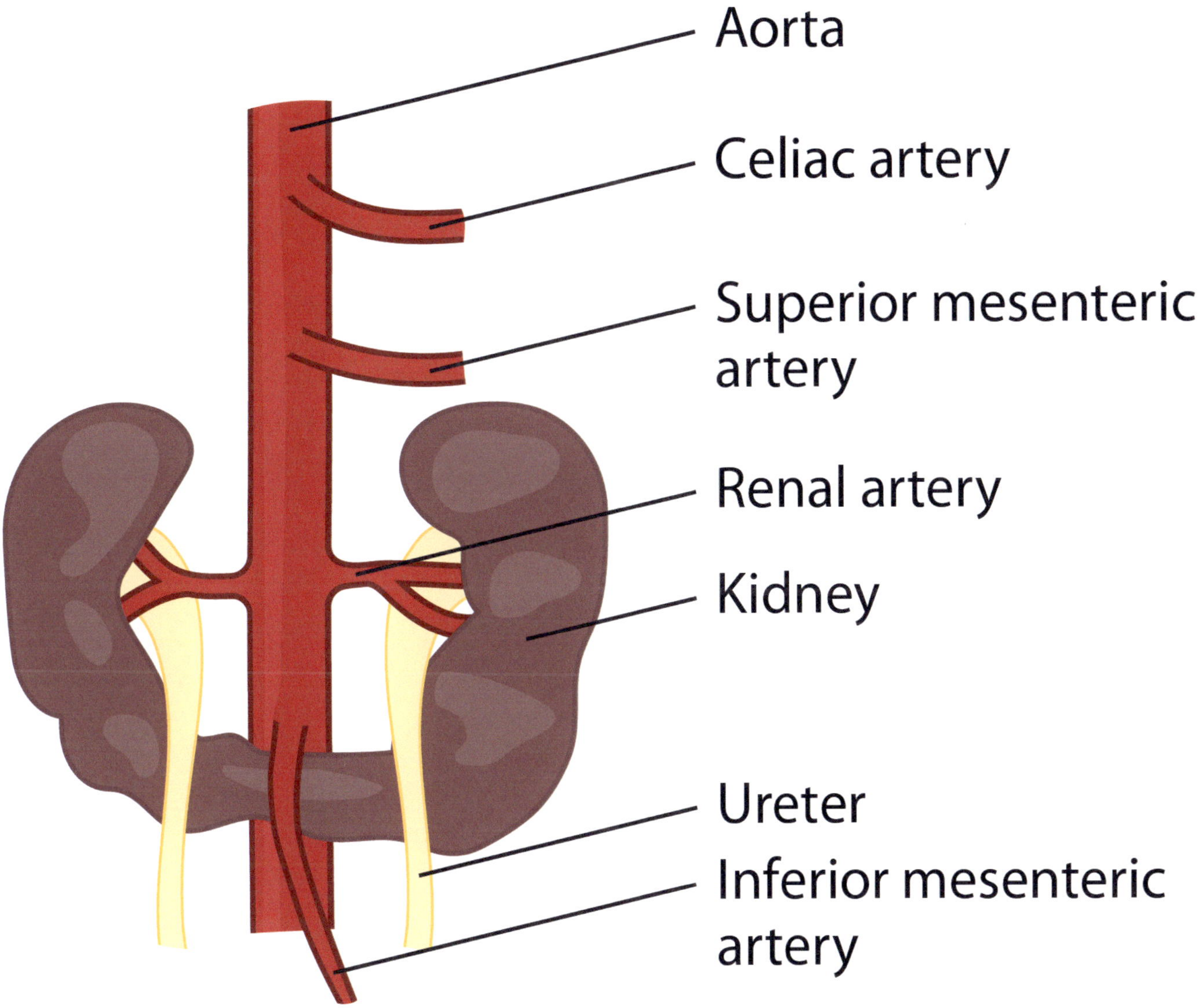

Figure 6.4.7 - Horseshoe kidney

REVIEW QUESTIONS

?

1. The connection between the left ureter and the left renal pelvis did not recanalize as normal. How will this abnormality most likely be manifest clinically?

- **Correct answer: infection of the left kidney**
- **What is being described here is ureteropelvic junction obstruction. This is most often a unilateral pathology, as in this patient with left-sided ureteropelvic junction obstruction**
- **Urine build-up → hydronephrosis → recurrent UTIs (eg, pyelonephritis)**
- **Example: a worried mother may bring her infant to the doctor because of fussiness and a fever (ie, the infant with this obstruction presented clinically with signs of infection)**

GASTROENTEROLOGY

Section I - Normal Gut Development

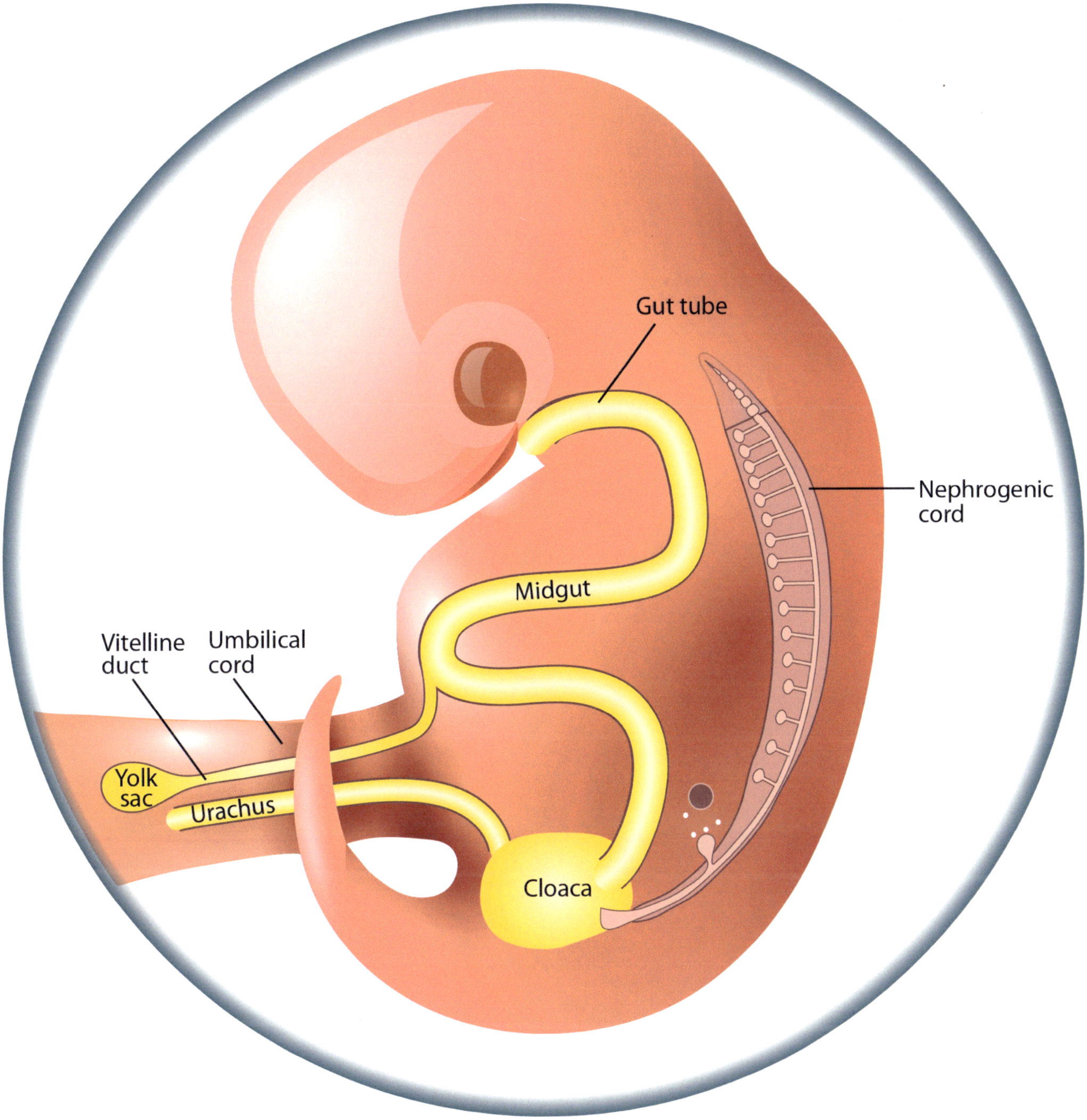

Figure 6.5.1 - Gut tube overview

I. Gastrointestinal Development

   A. Gut tube forms foregut, midgut and hindgut

   B. Yolk sac extends from the midgut through umbilical ring → vitelline duct connects midgut to yolk sac in the umbilical cord

   C. Midgut herniates into umbilical cord (week 5) → 90° counterclockwise rotation

   D. Midgut retracts into abdominal cavity (week 10) → 180° counterclockwise rotation (270° total)

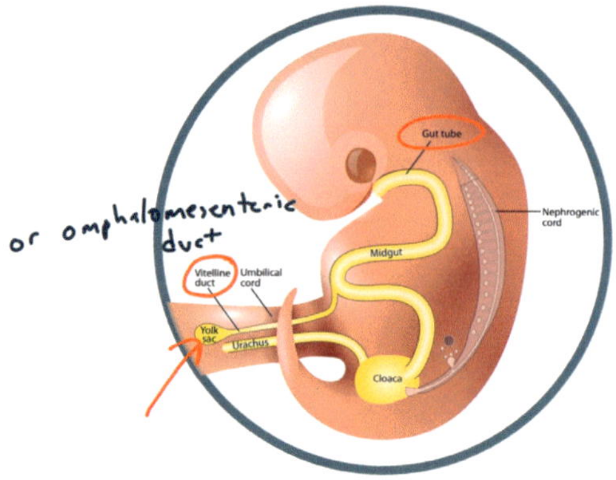

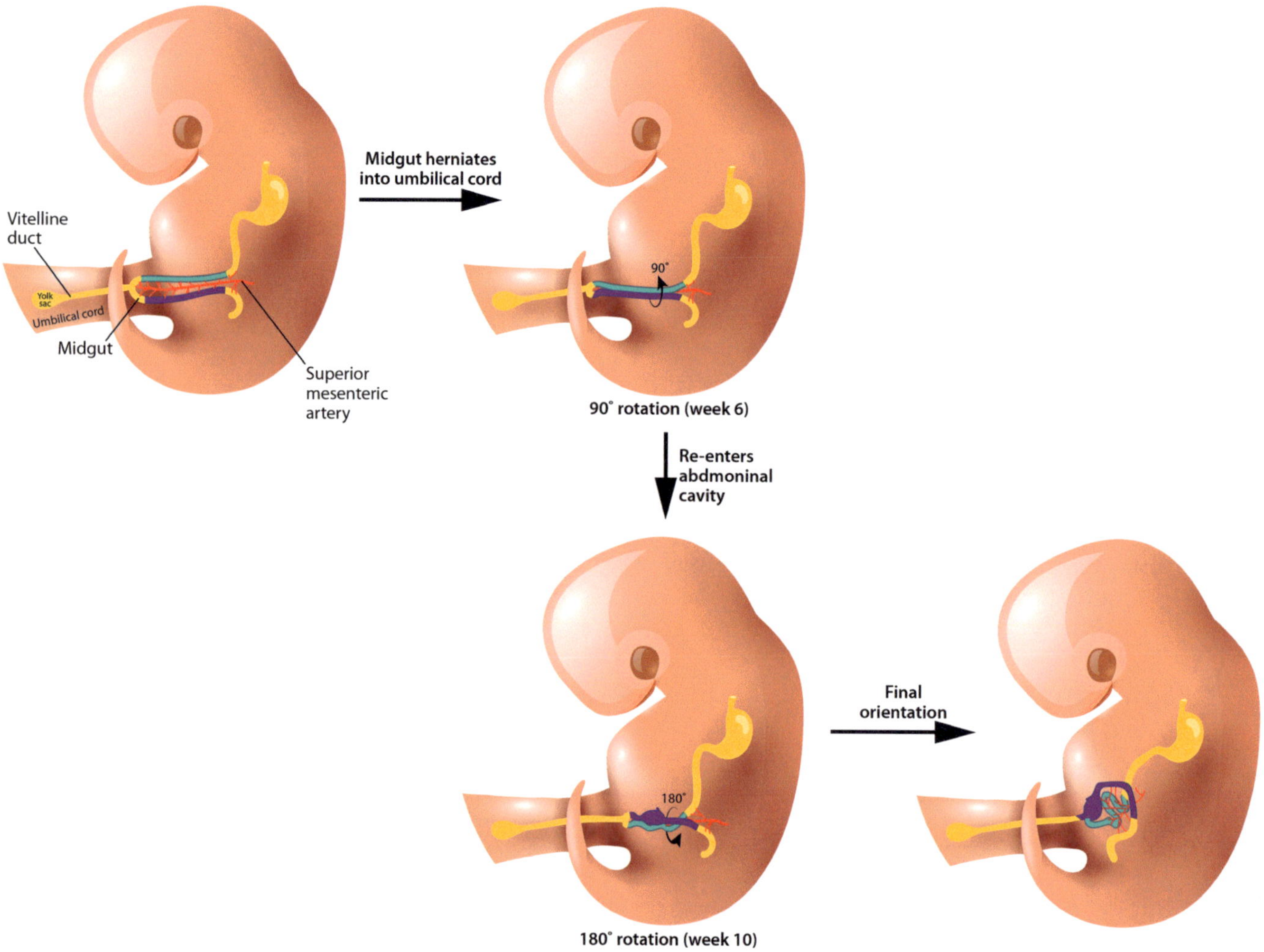

Figure 6.5.2 - Midgut rotation in utero

II. Gastrointestinal Divisions

A. Foregut

1. Esophagus to upper duodenum
2. Supplied by celiac trunk

B. Midgut

1. Lower duodenum to proximal ⅔ of transverse colon
2. Supplied by SMA

C. Hindgut

1. Distal ⅓ of transverse colon to anal canal above pectinate line
2. Supplied by IMA

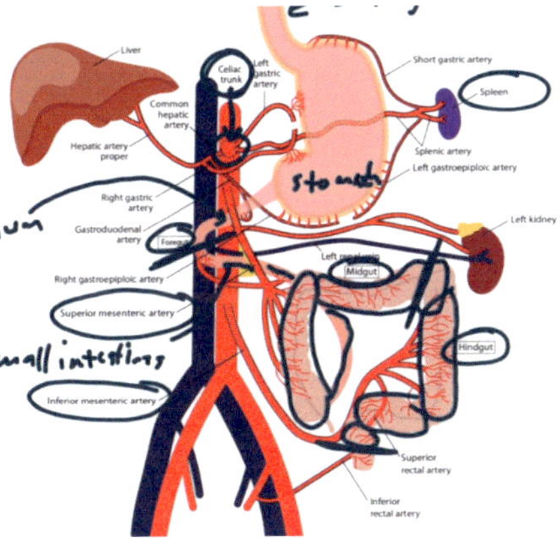

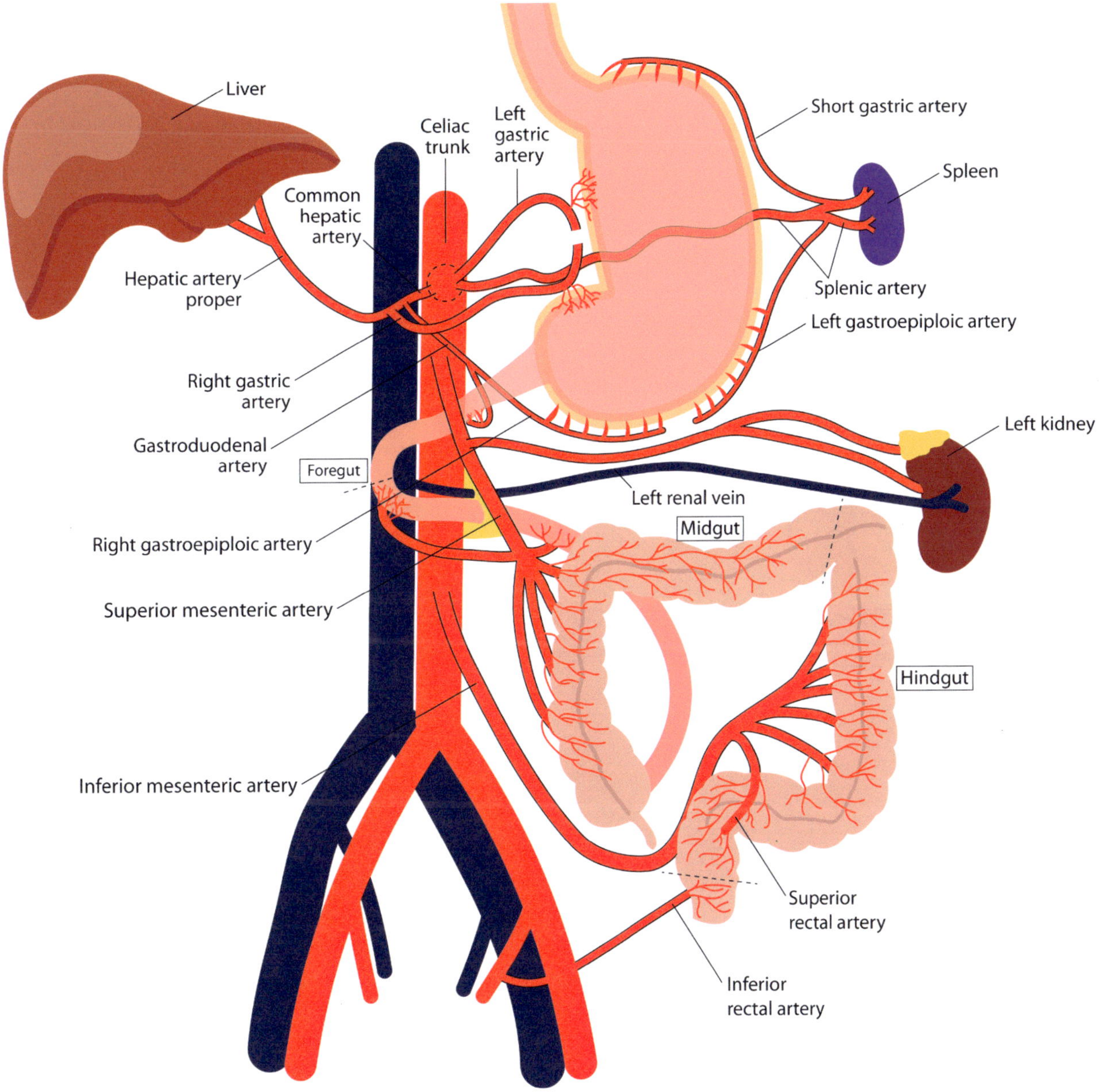

Figure 6.5.3 - Gastrointestinal arteries

REVIEW QUESTIONS ?

1. During fetal development, a portion of the gut tube herniates into the umbilical cord. This portion of the gut tube is supplied by a major artery that also supplies which of the following structures?

    A. Proximal duodenum
    B. Stomach
    C. Distal transverse colon
    D. Ascending colon

- **Correct answer: D**
- **The part of the gut tube that herniates into the umbilical cord is the midgut**
- **The midgut is supplied by the superior mesenteric artery**
- **The superior mesenteric also supplies the ascending colon**

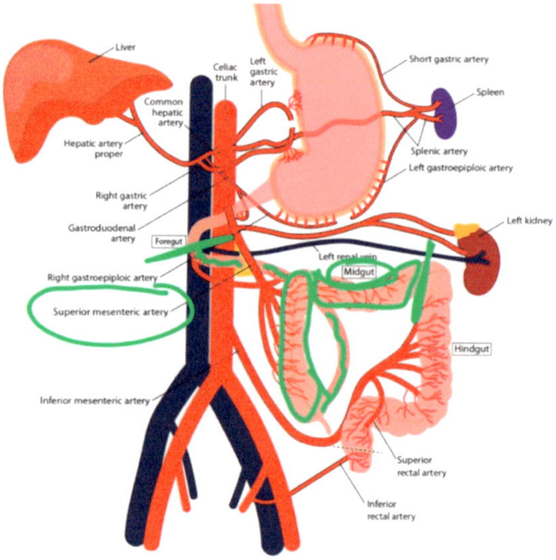

Section II - Pathology of Foregut and Hindgut Development

I. Hypertrophic Pyloric Stenosis

A. Pathophysiology

1. Hypertrophy of the inner circular layer → obstruction of the gastric outlet

B. Males (2-6 weeks old)

C. Presentation

1. Visible peristaltic waves
2. Olive-shaped mass
3. Nonbilious projectile vomiting → hypokalemic hypochloremic metabolic alkalosis (if vomiting > 3 weeks, uncommon)

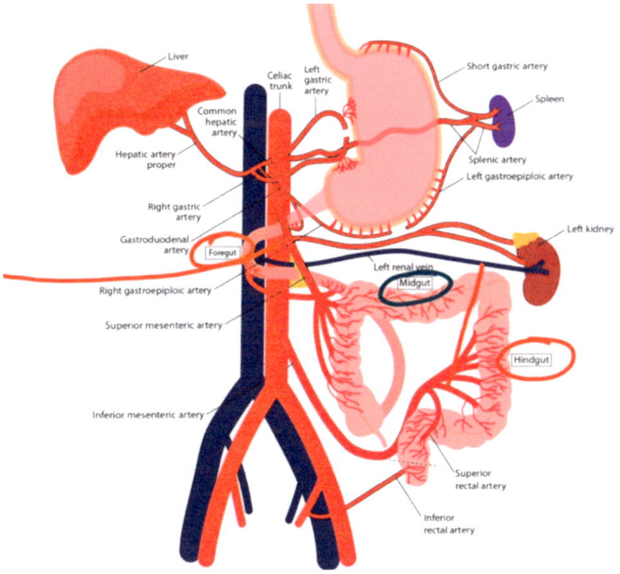

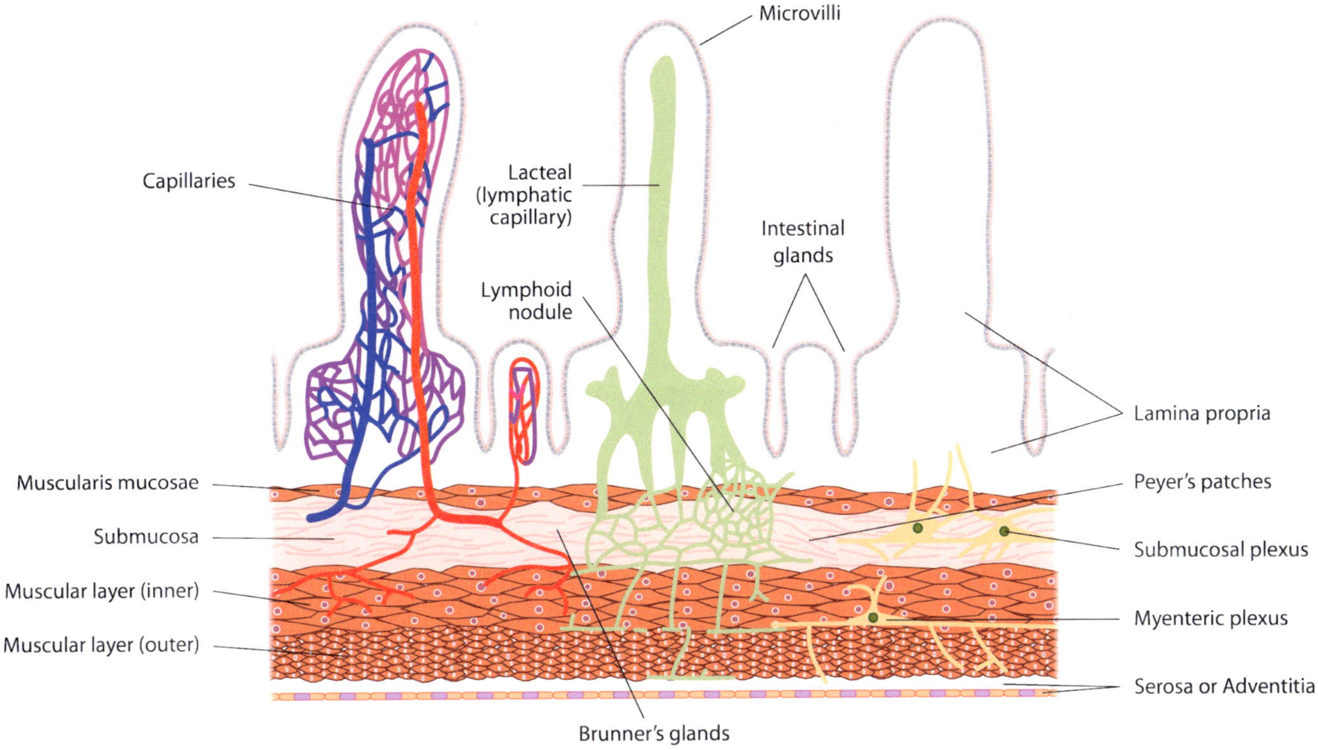

Figure 6.5.4 - Layers of the intestinal wall

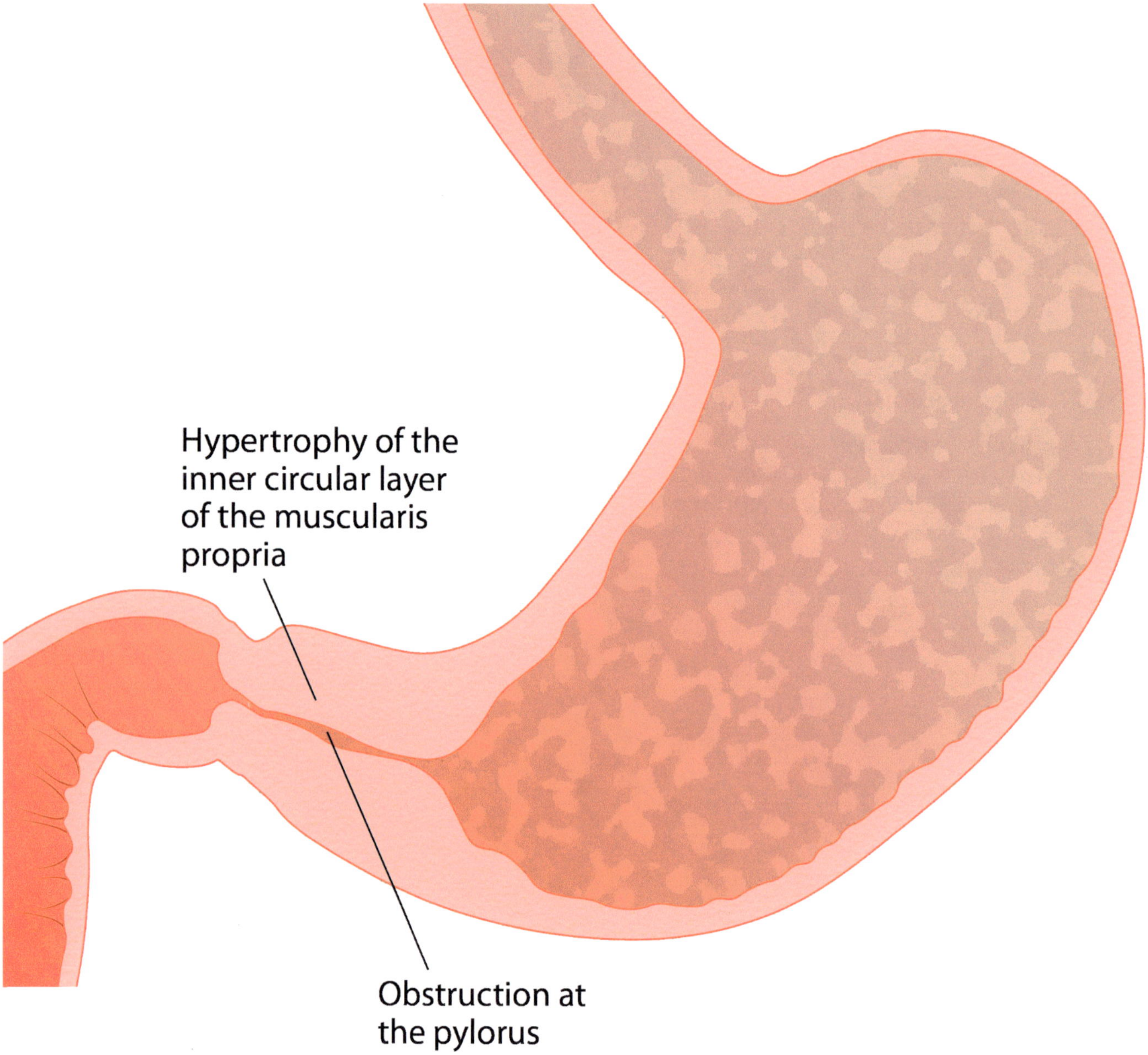

Figure 6.5.5 - Hypertrophic pyloric stenosis

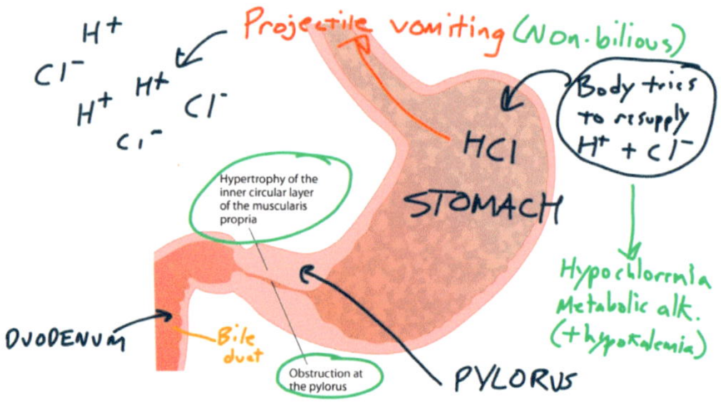

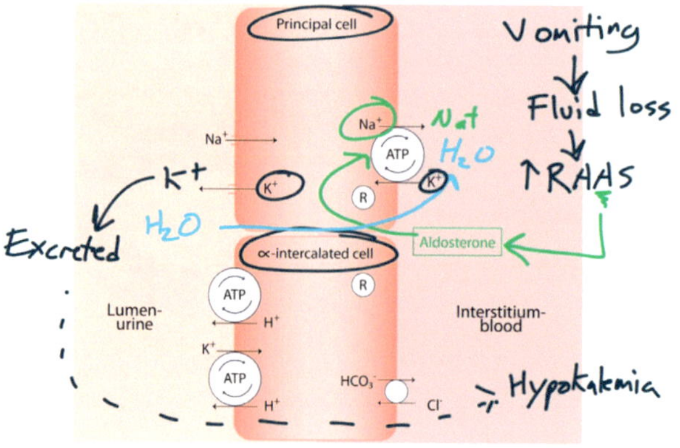

II. Hypertrophic Pyloric Stenosis: Risk Factors

   A. Maternal smoking

   B. Genetic factors

   C. Macrolide antibiotics

      1. Azithromycin

      2. Erythromycin

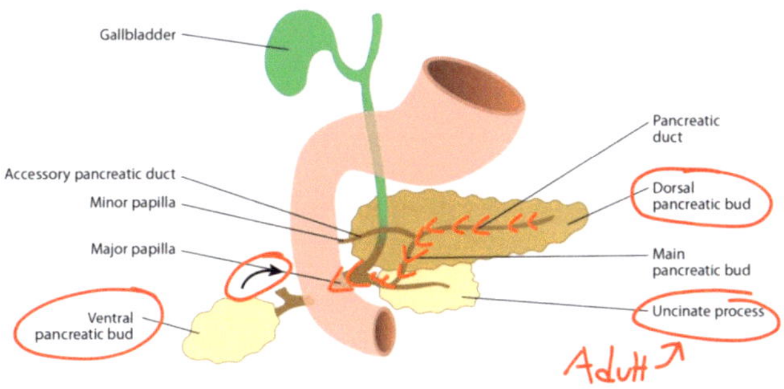

III. Pancreas Development

   A. Dorsal pancreatic bud

      1. Forms head, body, and tail

      2. Does not rotate

   B. Ventral pancreatic bud

      1. Sprouts into ventral mesentery

      2. Forms ventral pancreas, main pancreatic duct

      3. Rotates around duodenum

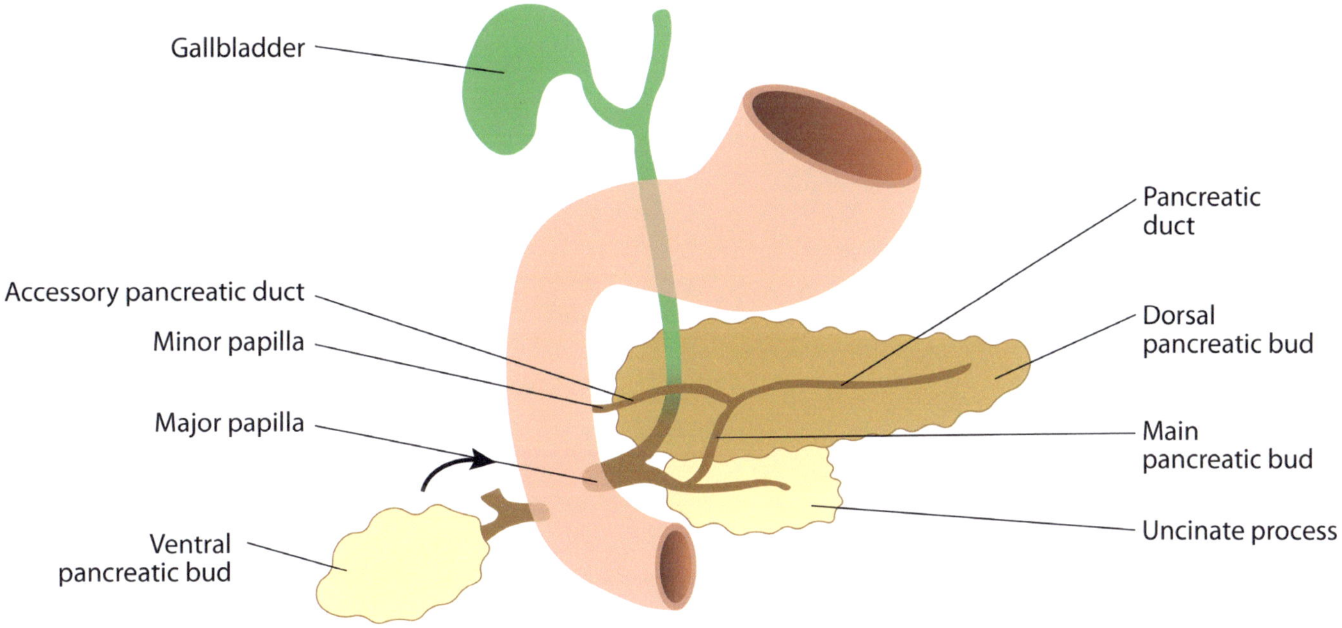

Figure 6.5.6 - Normal pancreatic rotation

IV. Pancreas Abnormalities

A. Annular pancreas

1. Failure of ventral bud to rotate or abnormal rotation of ventral bud
2. Forms ring around duodenum → narrowing → vomiting

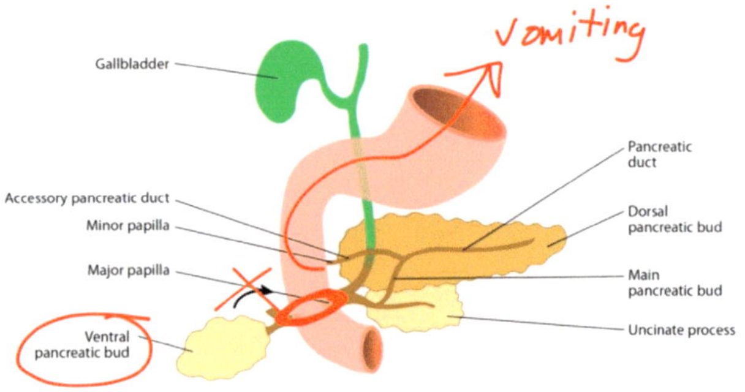

B. Pancreas divisum

1. Ventral and dorsal portions of duct system fail to fuse
2. Common
3. Occurs around week 8
4. Usually asymptomatic
5. Can lead to pancreatitis

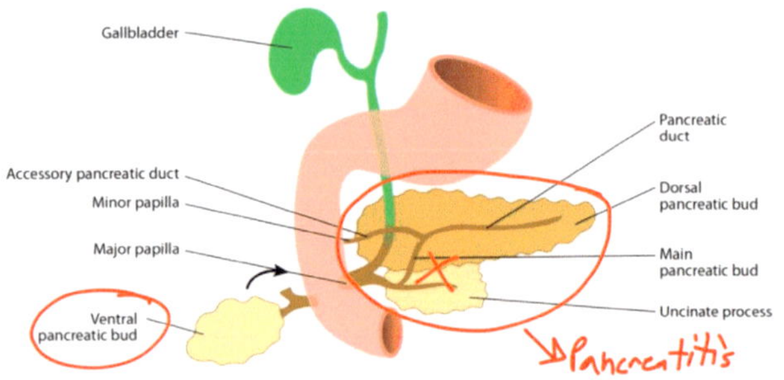

V. Spleen Development

A. Foregut vasculature (celiac trunk) also supplies spleen (splenic artery)

B. Develops from mesoderm (GI tract develops from all germ layers)

C. Site of hematopoiesis

D. Lymphatic organ by week 23

VI. Hirschsprung Disease

A. Motor disorder of the gut

1. Weeks 4-7
2. RET loss-of-function mutation

B. Defect in cranial-caudal migration of neuroblasts originating from neural crest cells

1. Aganglionic segment of gut fails to relax
2. Lack of ganglion cells/enteric nerve plexuses

C. Clinical Presentation:

1. Bilious emesis
2. Abdominal distension
3. Failure to pass meconium or stool in first 48 hours
4. Explosion of gas or stool upon digital exam of rectum

D. Treatment:

1. Bowel resection

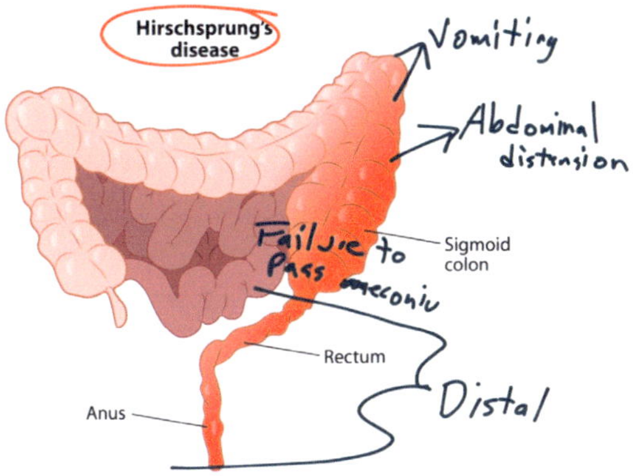

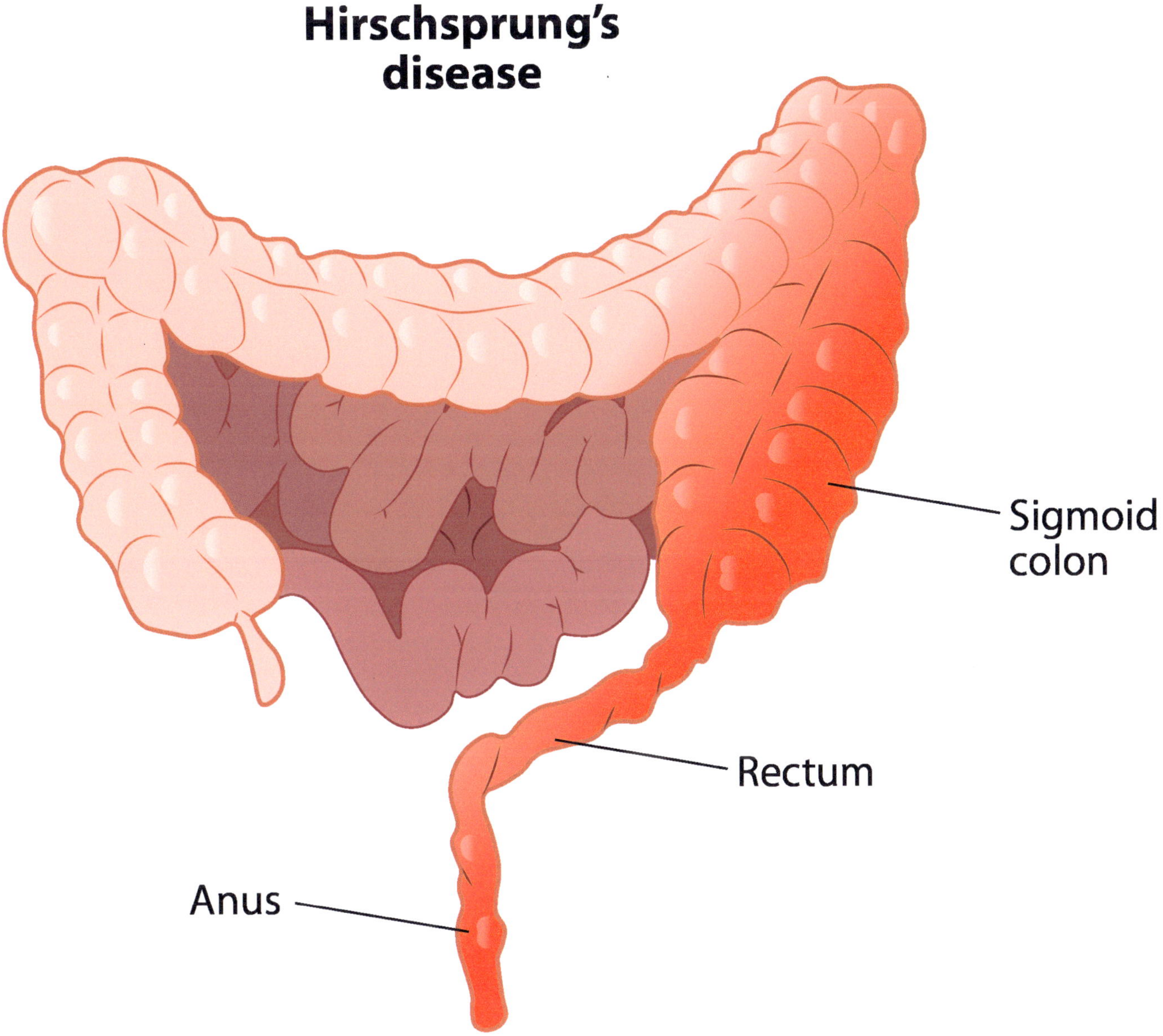

Figure 6.5.7 - Hirschsprung's disease

REVIEW QUESTIONS

1. During the development of a fetus, the ventral pancreatic bud rotates as normal, but fails to fuse with the dorsal bud. What is the most likely clinical outcome of this abnormality?

- **Correct answer: no symptoms**
- **Pancreas divisum occurs when the ventral bud rotates but fails to fuse with the dorsal bud**
- **Pancreas divisum is typically asymptomatic, but may cause pancreatitis**
- **Vomiting would be more consistent with an annular pancreas, in which the ventral bud fails to rotate as normal. That lack of rotation can form a ring around the duodenum and lead to obstruction**

Pancreas divisum
↓
Typically asymptomatic (pancreatitis possible)

Annular pancreas → Vomiting

Section III - Pathology of Midgut Development and Intestinal Atresia

I. Midgut Pathologies

  A. Meckel Diverticulum

  B. Congenital umbilical hernia

  C. Ventral wall defects (gastroschisis and omphalocele)

  D. Malrotation (duodenal obstruction and midgut volvulus)

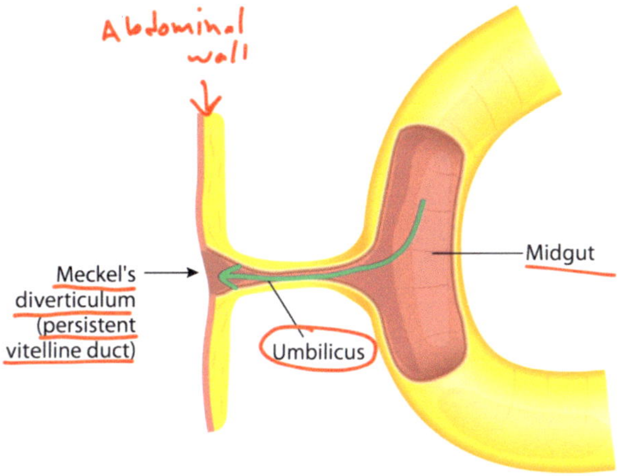

II. Meckel Diverticulum

  A. Results from incomplete obliteration of the vitelline (omphalomesenteric) duct

  B. Leads to formation of a true diverticulum

    1. Contains all three layers of the small bowel wall

  C. Can present with abdominal pain, or symptoms of GI bleeding or bowel obstruction

  D. Diagnosed by “Meckel scan”

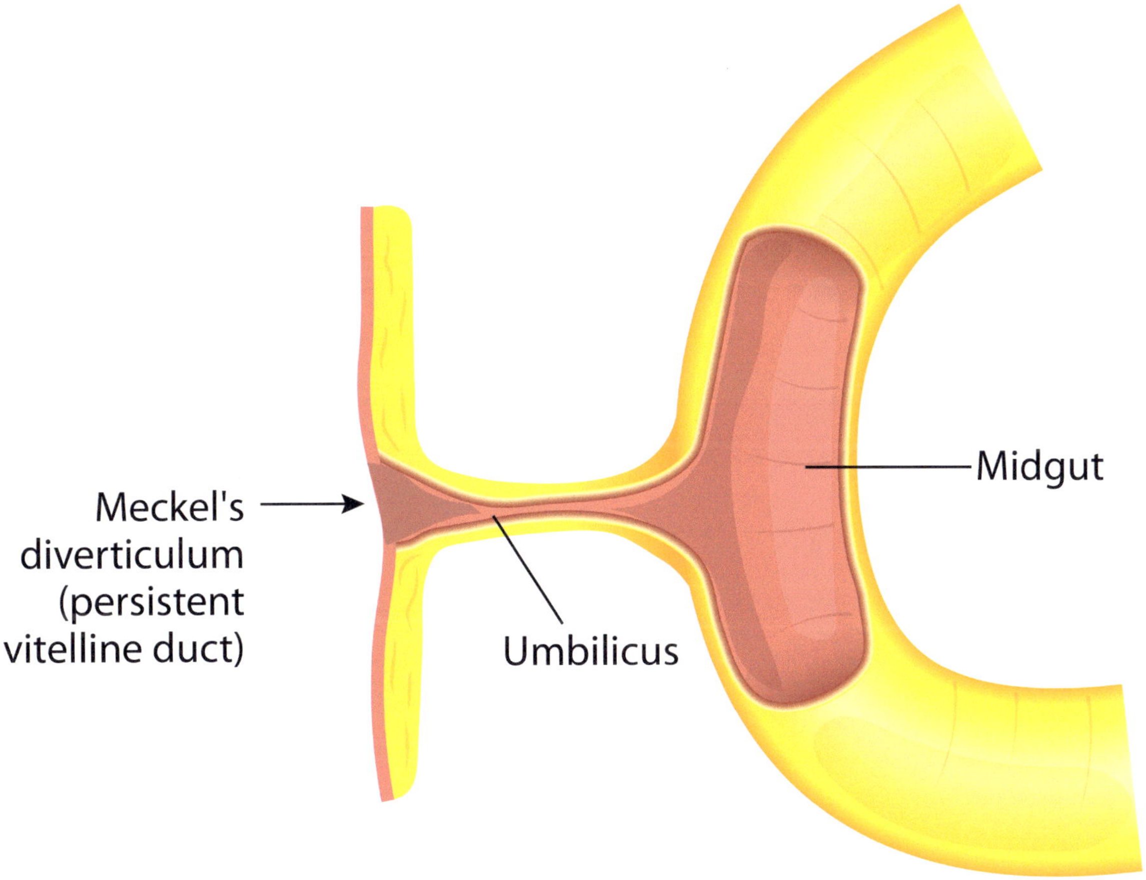

Figure 6.5.8 - Meckel diverticulum (lateral view)

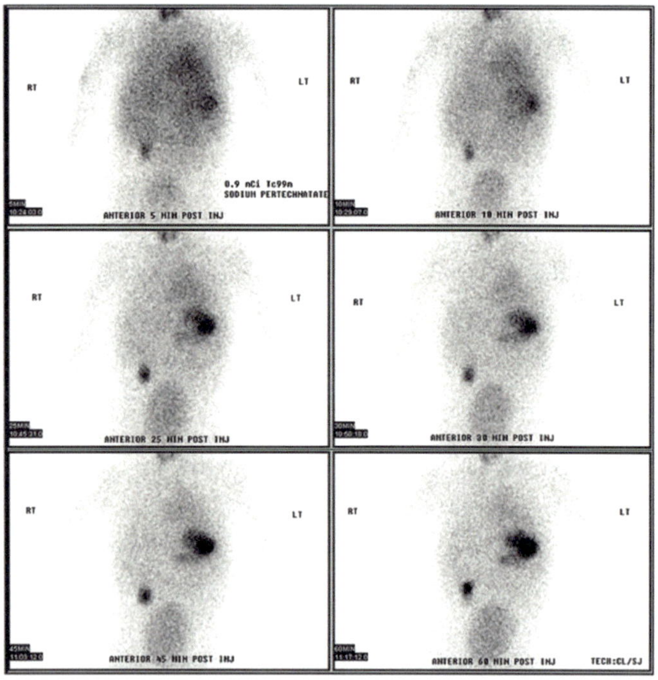

Photo Credit: JasonRobertYoungMD [CC BY-SA 4.0 (https://creativecommons.org/licenses/by-sa/4.0)]

Figure 6.5.9 - Meckel scan

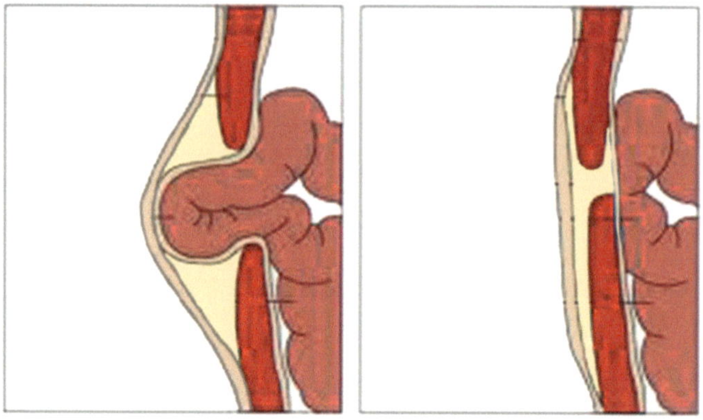

Figure 6.5.10 - Congenital umbilical hernia (lateral view)

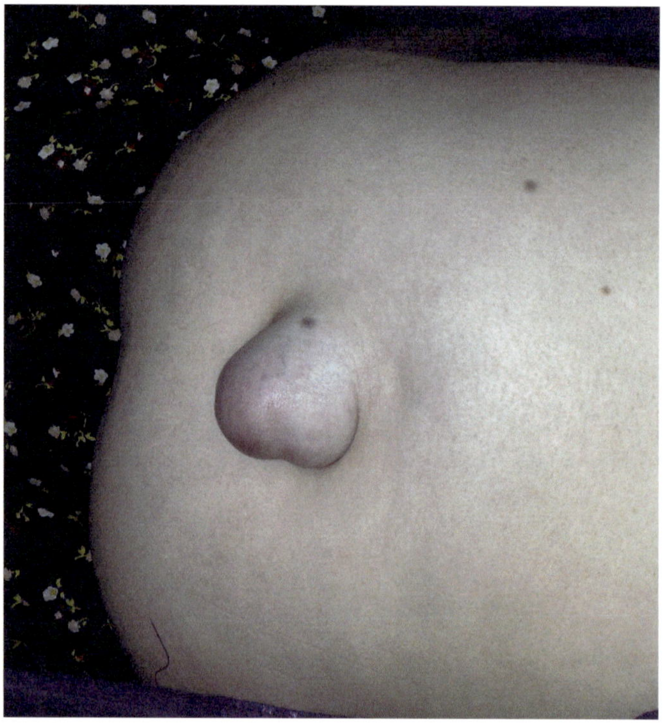

Photo Credit: Public Domain via Wiki

Figure 6.5.11 - Congenital umbilical hernia

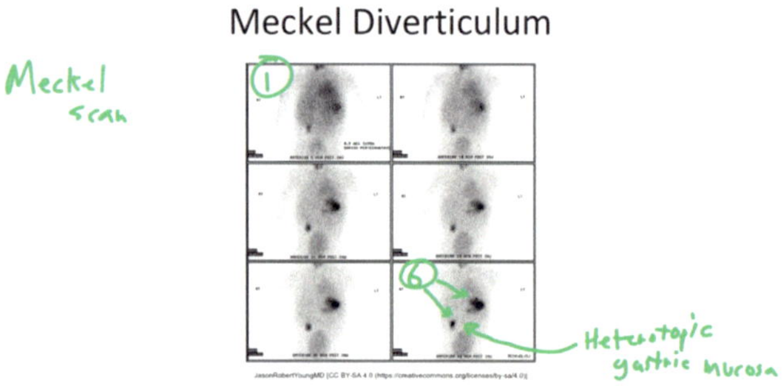

E. "Rule of 2's"

1. 2 times as likely in males
2. 2 inches long
3. 2 feet from the ileocecal valve
4. 2% of population
5. presents in first 2 years
6. may have 2 types of epithelia

III. Congenital Umbilical Hernia

A. Incomplete closure of the umbilical ring, allowing protrusion of bowel through the abdominal musculature

B. Soft, reducible, can cause pain in infant

C. Associated with Down syndrome

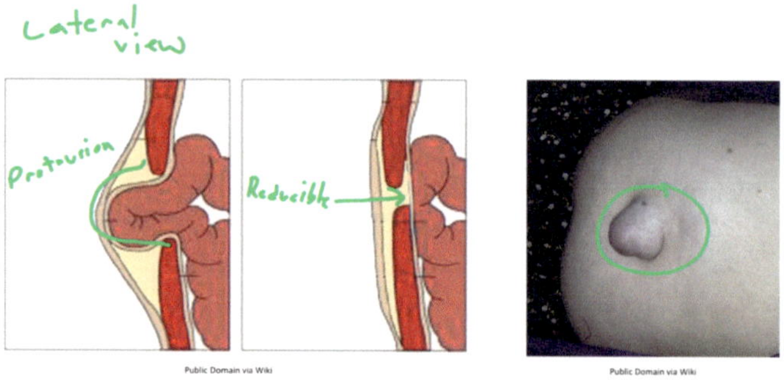

IV. Ventral Wall Defects

A. Gastroschisis

1. Defective formation or destruction of the body wall that results in herniation of abdominal contents through abdominal fold
2. No peritoneum covering
3. Usually right of midline
4. Few associated chromosome abnormalities

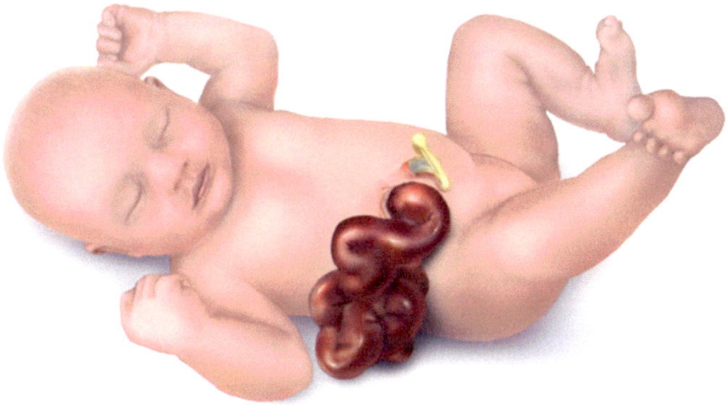

Photo Credit: Centers for Disease Control and Prevention

Figure 6.5.12 - Gastroschisis

B. Omphalocele

1. Abdominal wall defect in which lateral walls fail to migrate at the umbilical ring resulting in herniation of abdominal contents into umbilical cord
2. Peritoneal covering
3. Many associated chromosome abnormalities

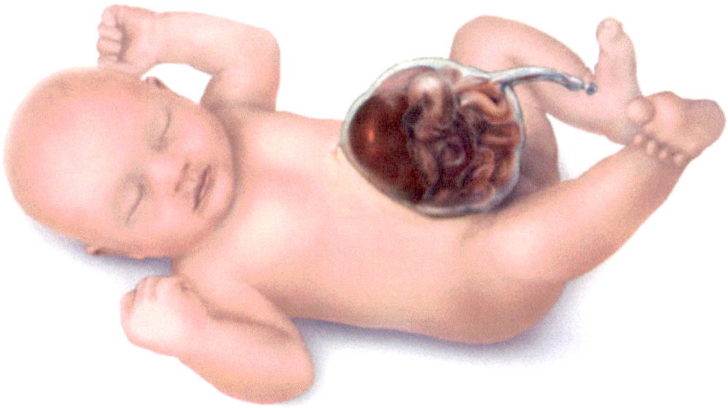

Photo Credit: Centers for Disease Control and Prevention

Figure 6.5.13 - Omphalocele

V. Midgut Malrotation

A. Arrest of normal rotation of embryonic gut tube → abnormal bowel positioning → Ladd bands and highly mobile small bowel

B. Potential consequences:

1. Duodenal obstruction
2. Midgut volvulus
3. Asymptomatic

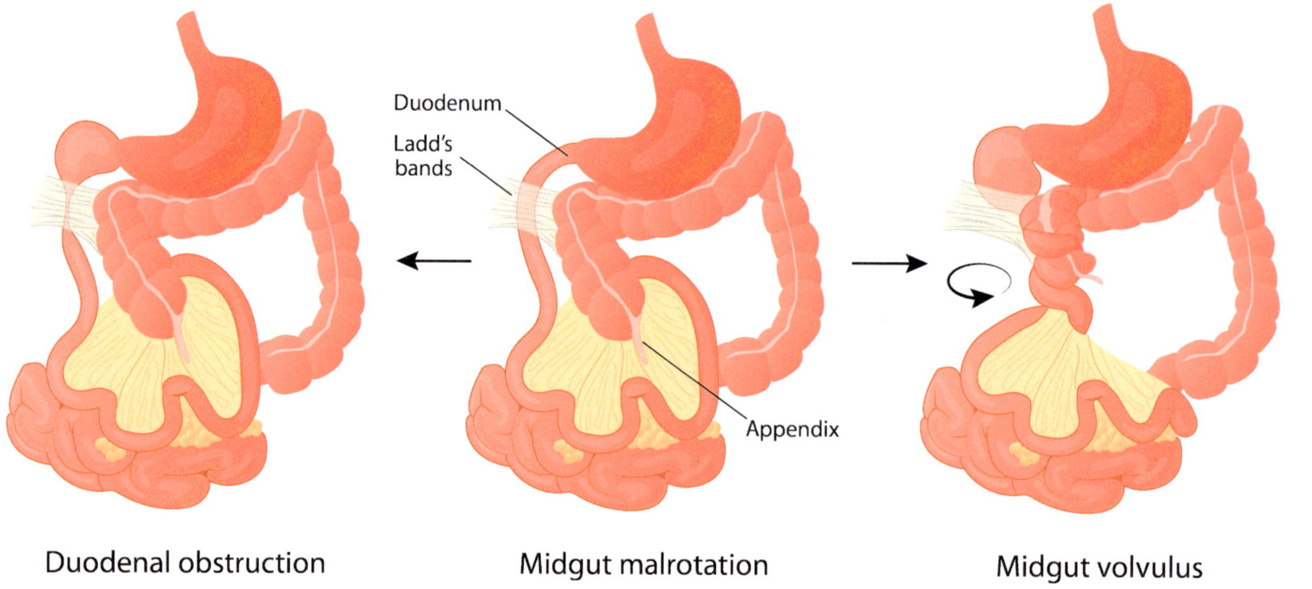

Figure 6.5.14 - Consequences of midgut malrotation

VI. Midgut Malrotation

A. Duodenal obstruction

1. Fibrous connective tissue from the peritoneum (Ladd bands) connect the proximal colon (often the cecum) to the right abdominal wall and cross the duodenum → extrinsic compression of duodenum → bilious vomiting and pain

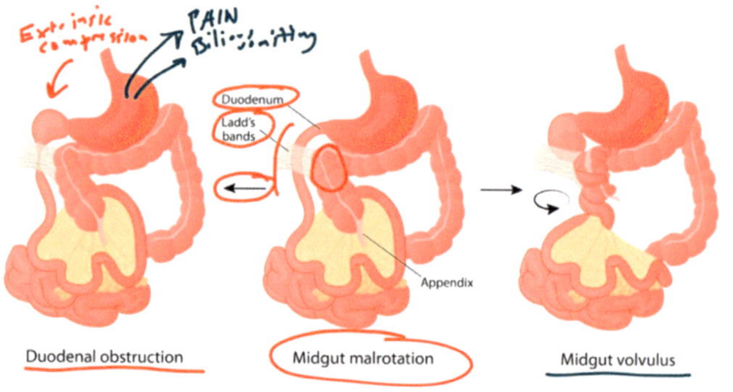

B. Midgut volvulus

1. Highly mobile small bowel → small bowel twists around mesentery

a) Early/mild consequences: small bowel obstruction → pain and bilious vomiting

b) Later/severe consequences: SMA occlusion → ischemic necrosis → perforation → septic shock and peritonitis (infection of peritoneum, rigid abdomen)

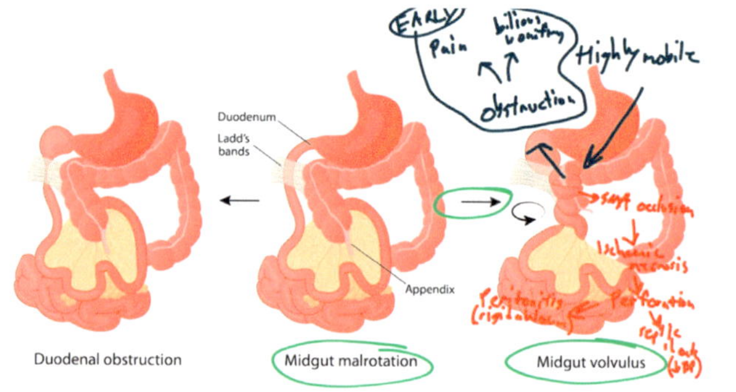

REVIEW QUESTIONS

1. A newborn experienced intestinal malrotation during development. Fibrous bands of connective tissue extend from the malpositioned cecum to the right abdominal wall. What symptom(s) might this newborn present with?

    - **Correct answer: bilious vomiting and abdominal distension**
    - **Fibrous bands of connective tissue (Ladd bands) can cause extrinsic compression of the duodenum**
    - **Duodenal obstruction can cause bilious vomiting and abdominal distension.**

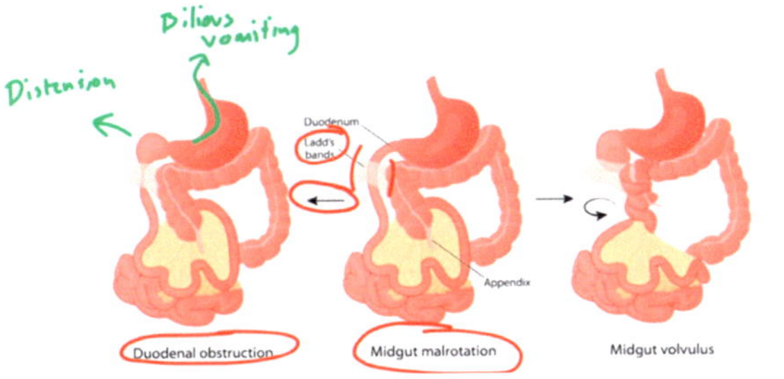

Section IV - Intestinal Atresia

I. Duodenal Atresia

A. Duodenal atresia (failure to recanalize duodenum distal to pylorus and common bile duct)

B. Associated with Down syndrome in 30% of cases

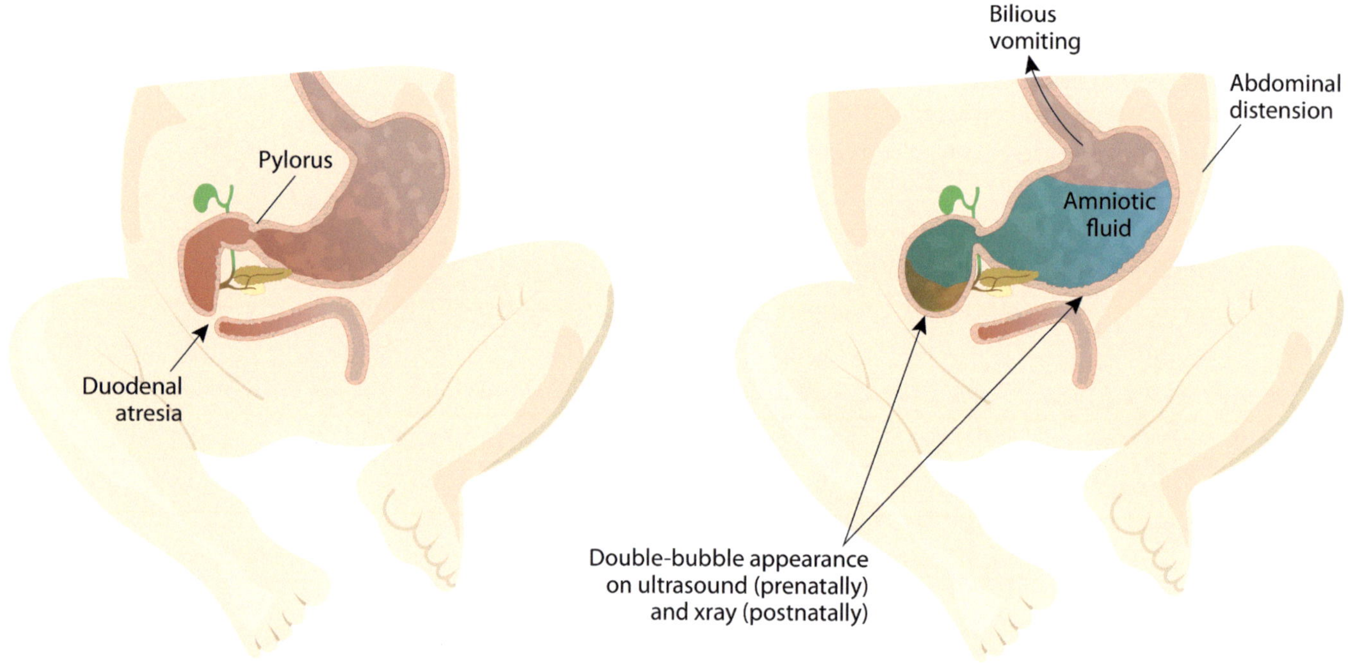

Figure 6.5.15 - Duodenal atresia

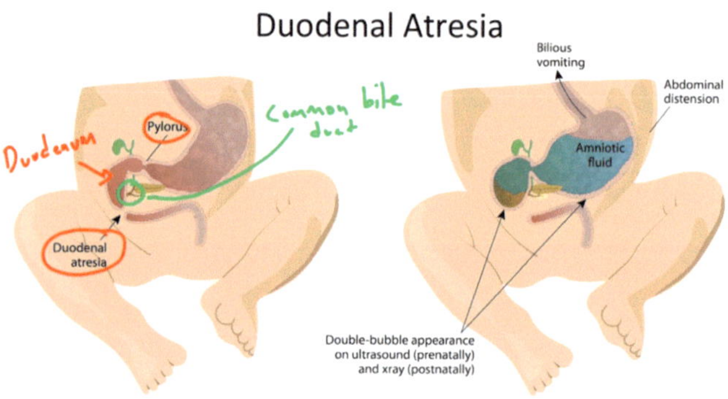

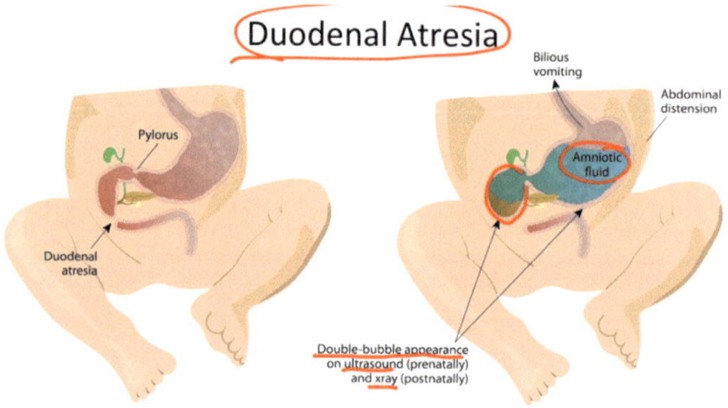

C. Prenatal findings

1. Failure to swallow sufficient amniotic fluid → polyhydramnios
2. Amniotic fluid distal to pylorus → double-bubble on ultrasound

D. Postnatal findings

1. Amniotic fluid distal to pylorus → double-bubble on x-ray
2. Amniotic fluid cannot pass duodenum → abdominal distension
3. Bile cannot pass duodenum → bilious vomiting

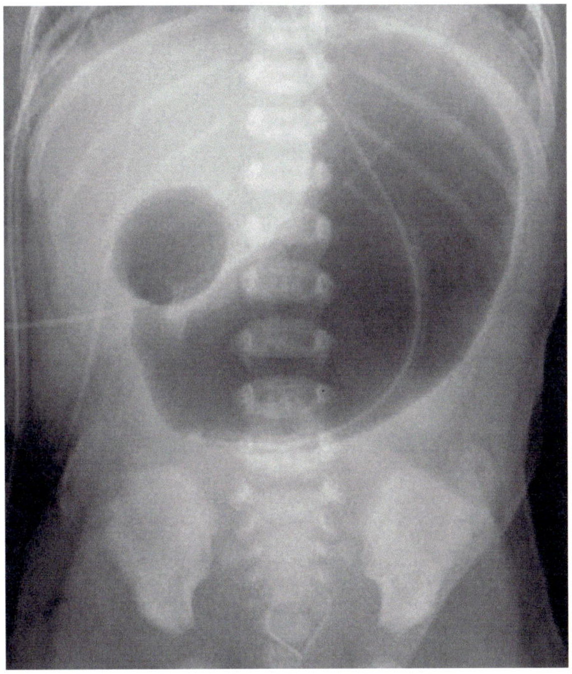

Photo Credit: Kinderradiologie Olgahospital Klinikum Stuttgart

Figure 6.5.16 - Double bubble sign on radiograph

II. Jejunal and Ileal Atresia

A. Jejunal and ileal atresia (SMA occlusion → ischemic bowel necrosis)

B. Prenatal findings

1. Failure to swallow sufficient amniotic fluid → polyhydramnios

C. Postnatal findings

1. Swallowed amniotic fluid builds up proximal to atresia → abdominal distension

2. Bile cannot pass through small intestines → bilious vomiting

3. Distal bowel spirals around a small branch of the SMA → apple-peel appearance (x-ray or during surgery)

Jejunal and Ileal Atresia

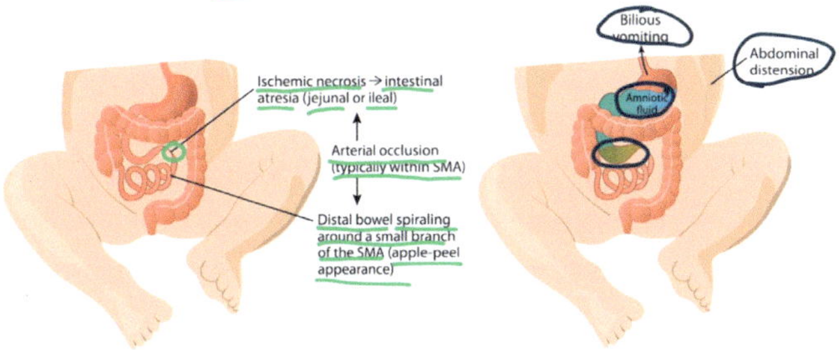

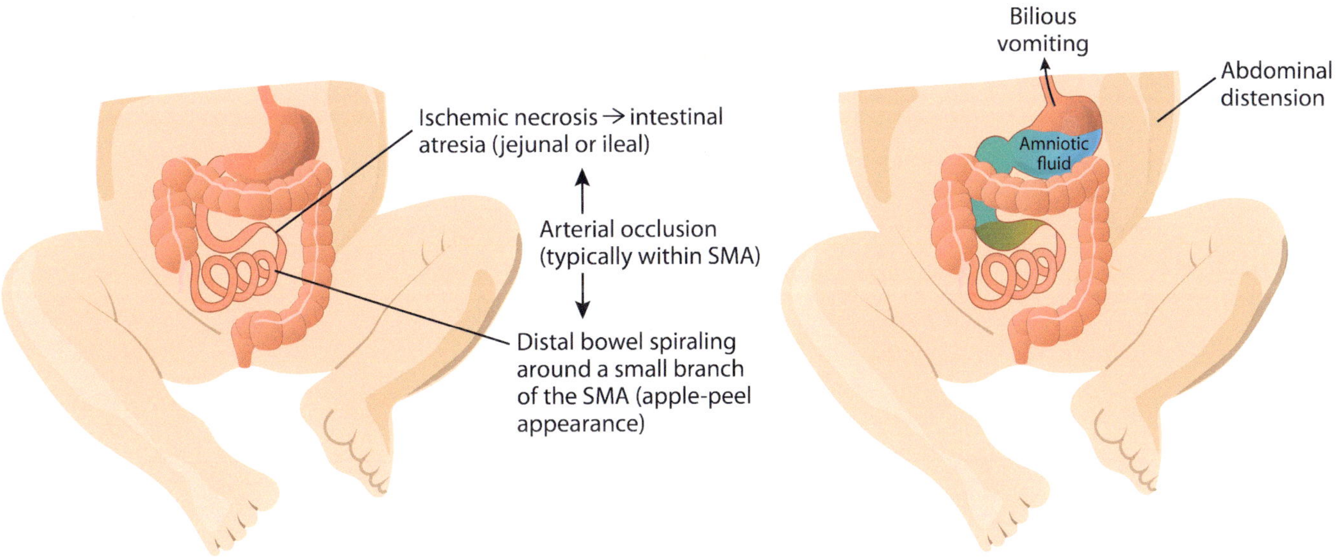

Figure 6.5.17 - Jejunal and Ileal Atresia

REVIEW QUESTIONS

1. A newborn demonstrates bilious vomiting and abdominal distension. Imaging reveals a second "bubble" just distal to an enlarged stomach. In utero, did this newborn more likely experience ischemic bowel necrosis or failure to recanalize a portion of the small intestines?

- **Correct answer: failure to recanalize a portion of the small bowel**
- **The stem describes the double bubble sign which indicates duodenal atresia**
- **Duodenal atresia occurs because the duodenum fails to recanalize**
- **Jejunal and ileal atresia occur because of SMA occlusion which leads to ischemic bowel necrosis**

Failure of recanalization
↓
Duodenal Atresia
↓
"Double bubble"

SMA occlusion → Ischemic necrosis
↓
Jejunal/Ileal Atresia

ENDOCRINOLOGY

Section I - Endocrine Embryology

I. Endocrine Embryology
   A. Thyroid gland
   B. Pituitary gland

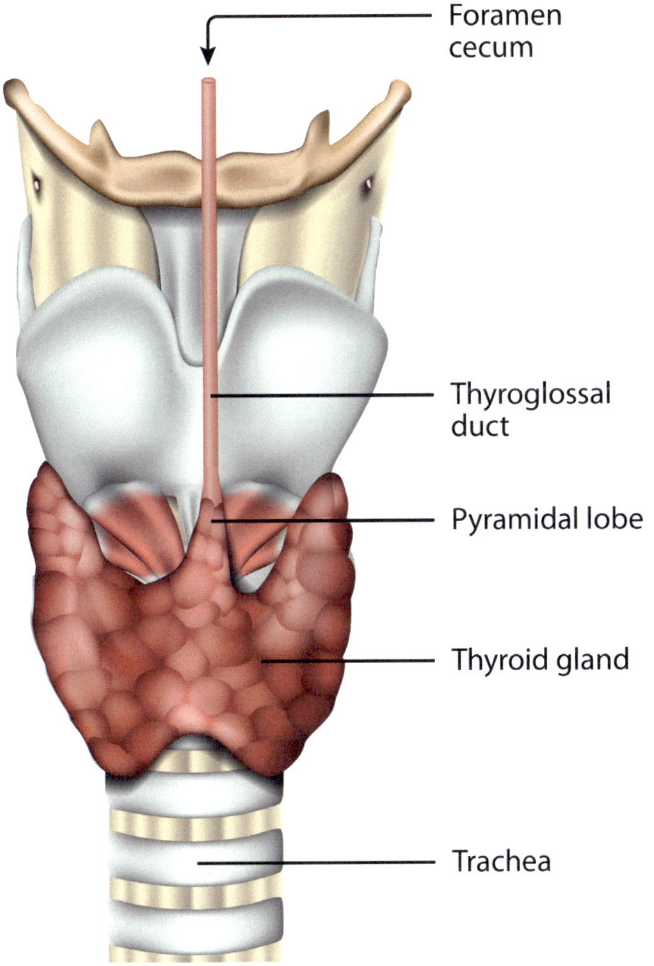

Figure 6.6.1 - Anterior view of the thyroid

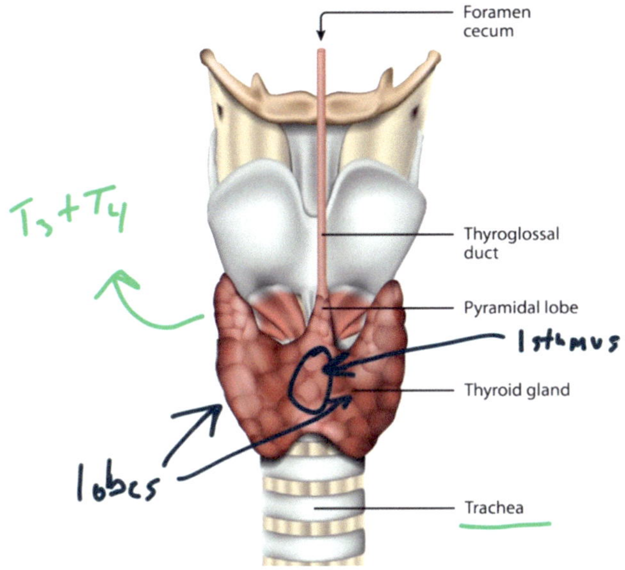

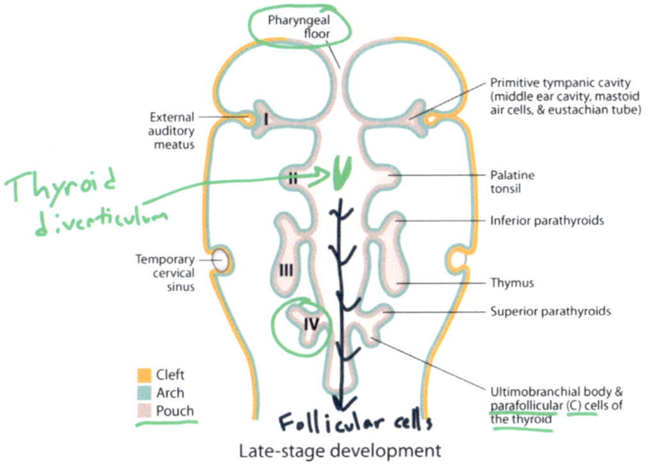

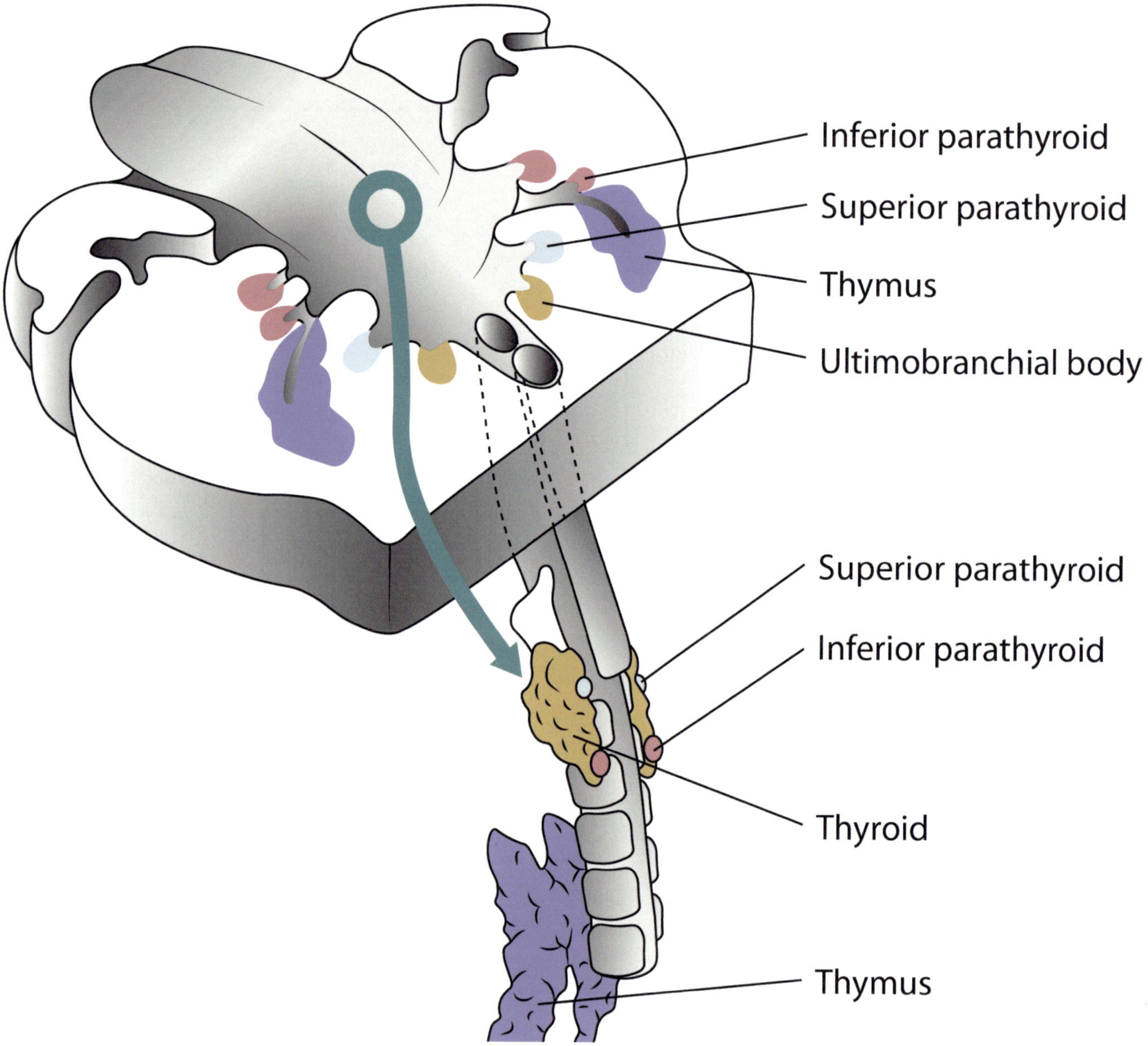

Figure 6.6.2 - Descent of thyroid during development

II. Thyroid Gland Embryology

A. Thyroid diverticulum travels from pharyngeal apparatus down to form the thyroid gland → thyroid tissue (follicular and parafollicular cells) are derived from endoderm

B. Thyroglossal duct is the pathway between the thyroid and tongue → degenerates

III. Thyroglossal Duct Remnants

A. Thyroglossal duct degenerates → some structures persist

B. Normal

1. Foramen cecum

2. Pyramidal lobe

C. Abnormal

1. Thyroglossal duct → can lead to thyroglossal duct cysts

IV. Thyroglossal Duct Cyst

A. Failure of thyroglossal duct to degenerate

1. Midline

2. Moveable mass

3. Asymptomatic

4. Seen by 5 years of age

5. May or may not have thyroid tissue

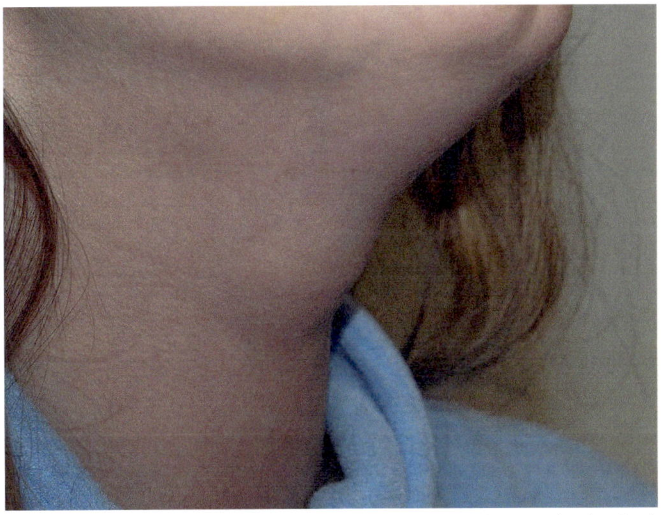

Figure 6.6.3 - Thyroglossal duct cyst

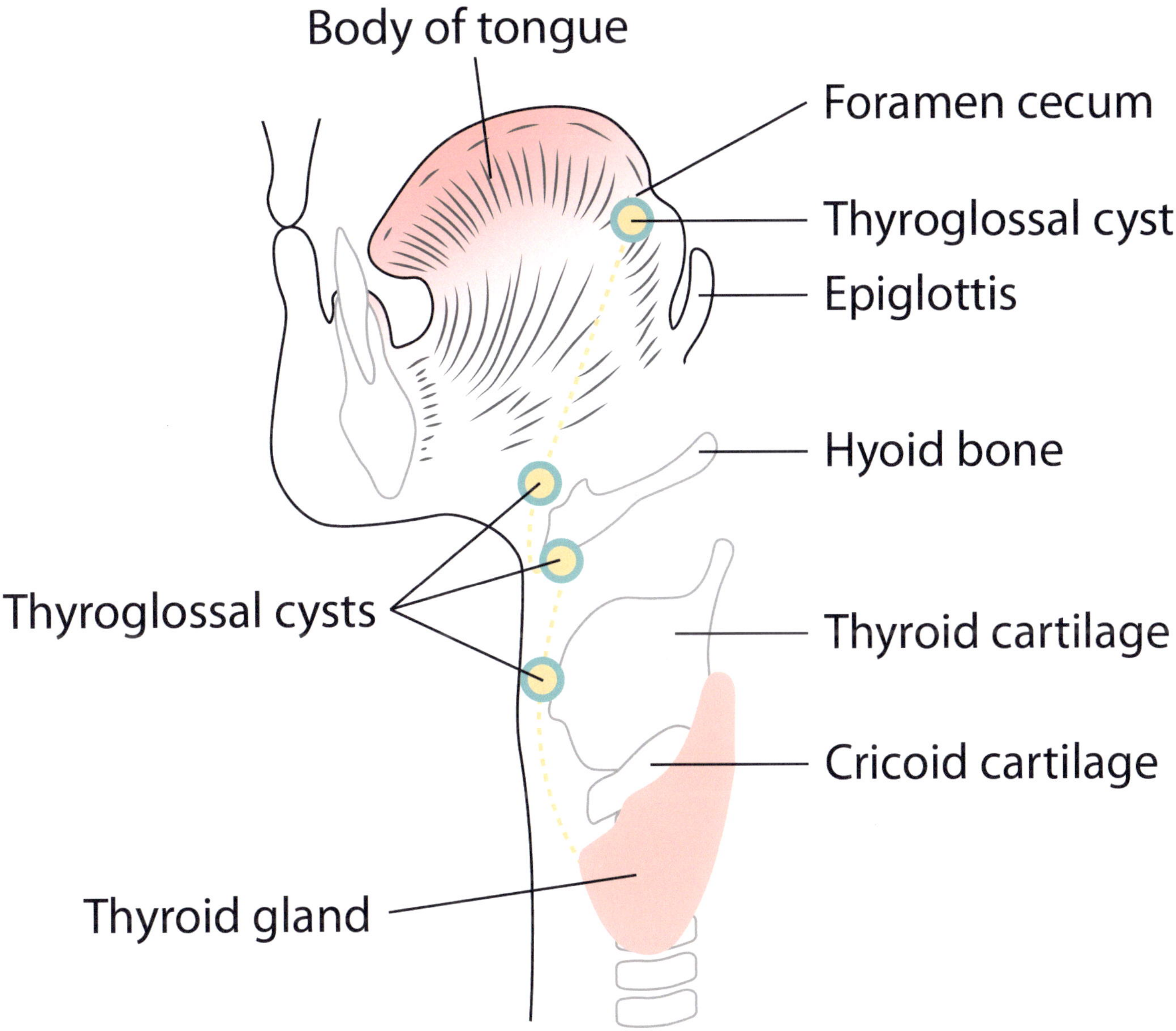

Figure 6.6.4 - Possible locations of thyroglossal duct cysts

V. Ectopic Thyroid

A. Thyroid tissue found in abnormal places

1. Most common site is the tongue
2. Removal may cause hypothyroidism

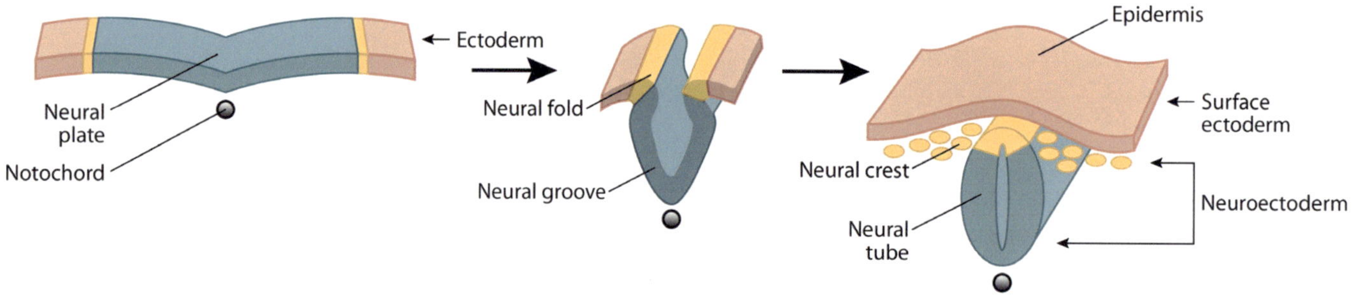

Figure 6.1.10 - Neurulation

VI. Pituitary Gland Embryology

A. Posterior pituitary

1. Neuroectoderm from diencephalon → connected to hypothalamus

B. Anterior pituitary

1. Surface ectoderm from roof of mouth → forms Rathke's pouch
2. Craniopharyngioma is a remnant of Rathke's pouch

VII. Posterior Pituitary

A. ADH and oxytocin are made in the hypothalamus

B. Released from the posterior pituitary

VIII. Pituitary Gland Embryology

A. Posterior pituitary

1. Forms from the neuroectoderm of the diencephalon → connected to hypothalamus

B. Anterior pituitary

1. Forms from the surface ectoderm of the roof of the mouth → forms Rathke's pouch
2. Craniopharyngioma is a remnant of Rathke's pouch

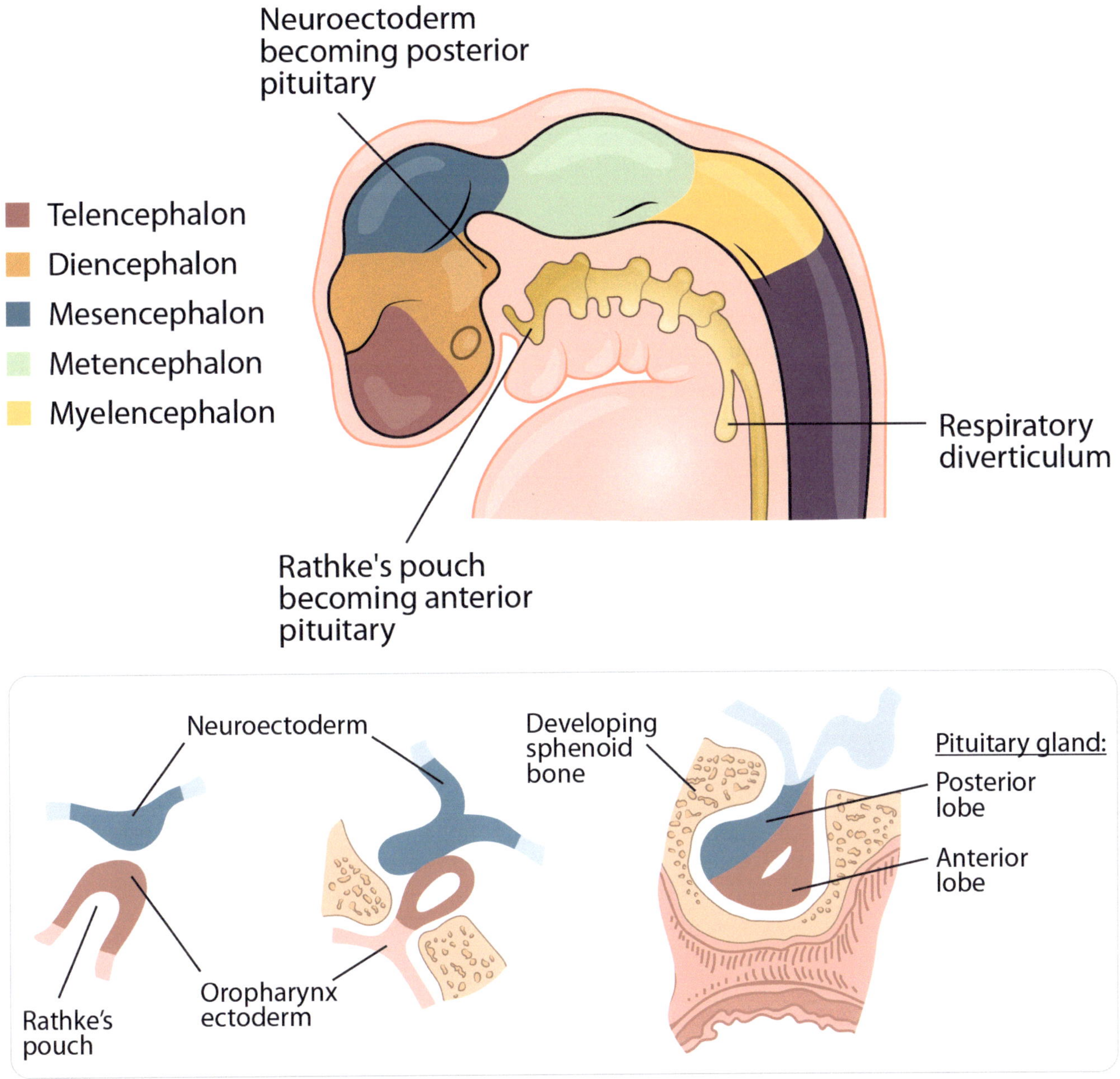

Figure 6.6.5 - Formation of the pituitary gland

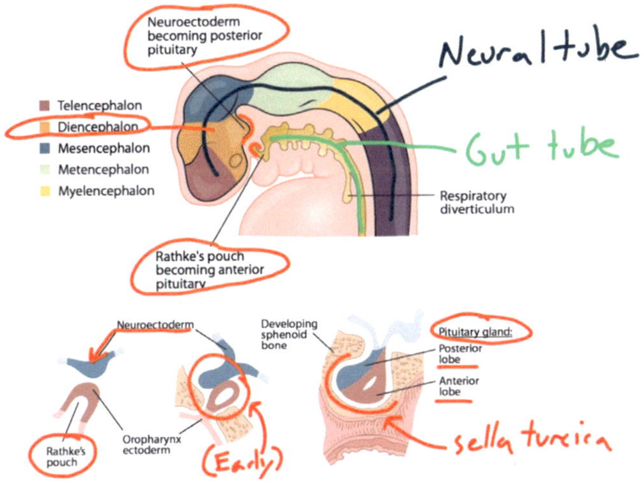

REVIEW QUESTIONS

1. A gland derived from the endoderm is dysfunctional. Which hormone was most likely released by this gland: ADH or triiodothyronine?

- **Answer: triiodothyronine**
- **Triiodothyronine (T_3) is released from the thyroid gland which originated from the endoderm of the pharyngeal apparatus**
- **ADH is released from the posterior pituitary gland which is derived from neuroectoderm (from ectoderm)**

A gland derived from the endoderm is dysfunctional. Which hormone was most likely released by this gland: ADH or triiodothyronine?

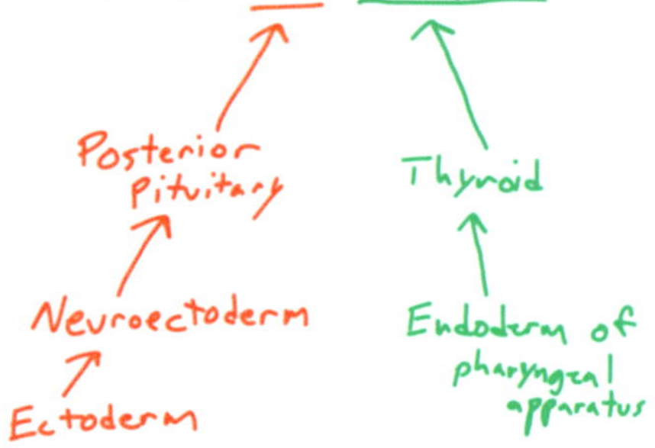

NEUROLOGY

Section I - Neurulation and Neural Tube Defects

I. Germ Layer Origins

A. Ectoderm

1. Surface ectoderm: anterior pituitary, lens, cornea
2. Neuroectoderm
    a) Neural tube: spinal cord, brain, posterior pituitary, retina
    b) Neural crest: skull, autonomic, sensory nerves

II. Neurulation

A. Occurs between day 18-21

B. Notochord signals formation of neural plate

C. Neural plate is folded and becomes 2 important components

1. Neural tube
2. Neural crest cells

D. Notochord becomes nucleus pulposus

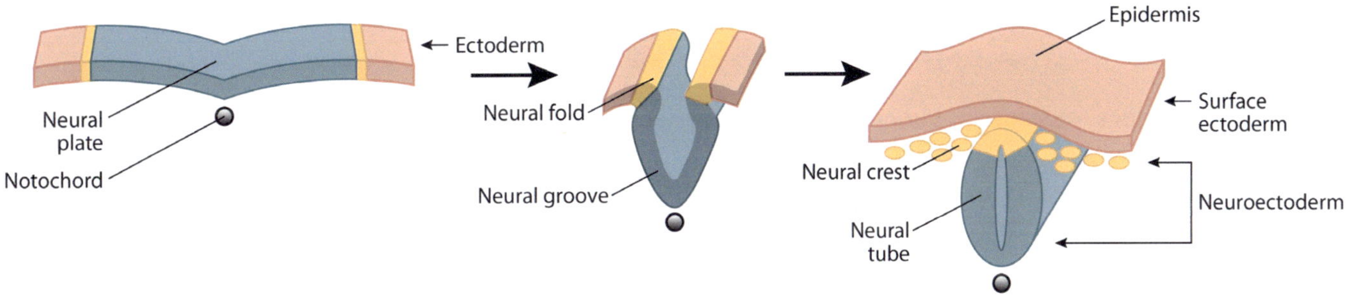

Figure 6.1.10 - Neurulation

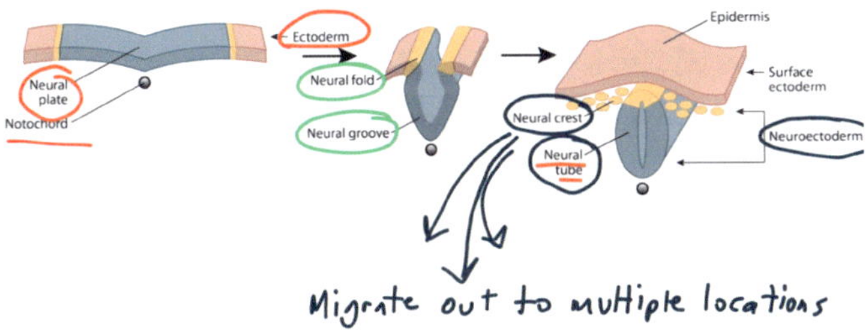

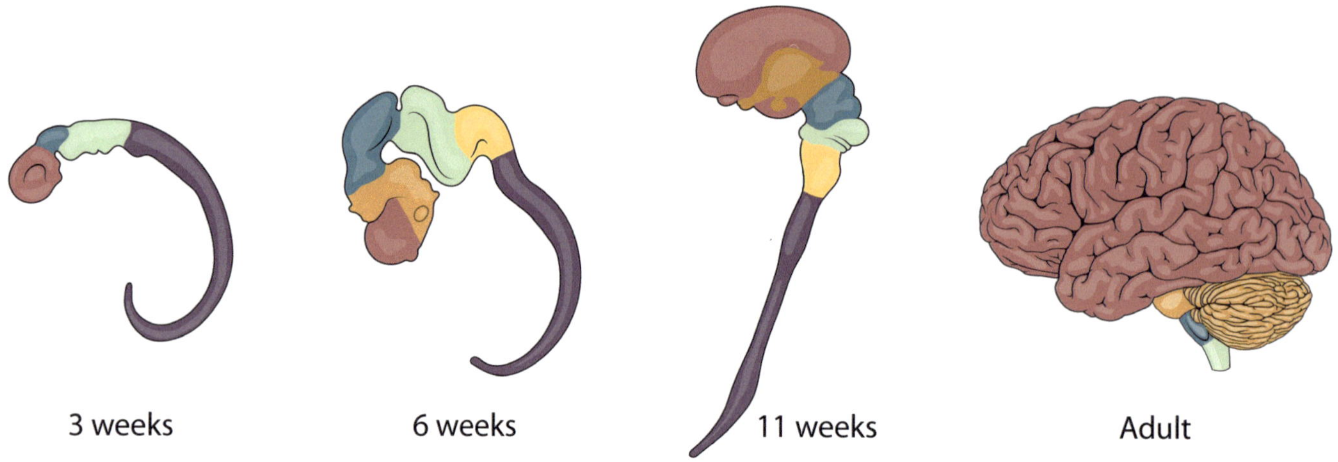

Figure 6.7.1 - Lateral view of neural tube progression

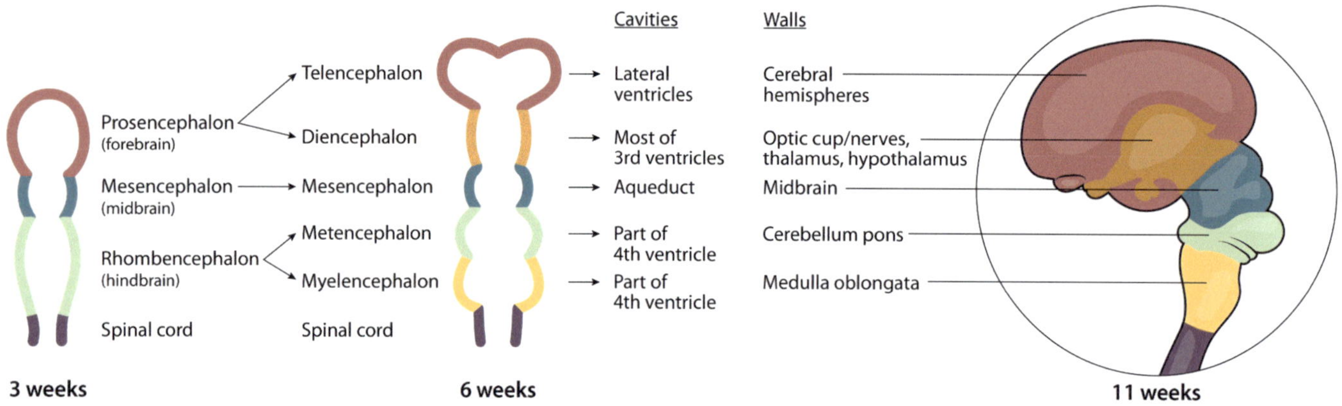

Figure 6.1.6 - Brain segments, cavities and walls derived from the neural tube

III. Neural Tube Defects

A. Neuropore should fuse by week 4

B. Fusion failure → persistent connection between amniotic cavity and spinal canal (neural tube defect)

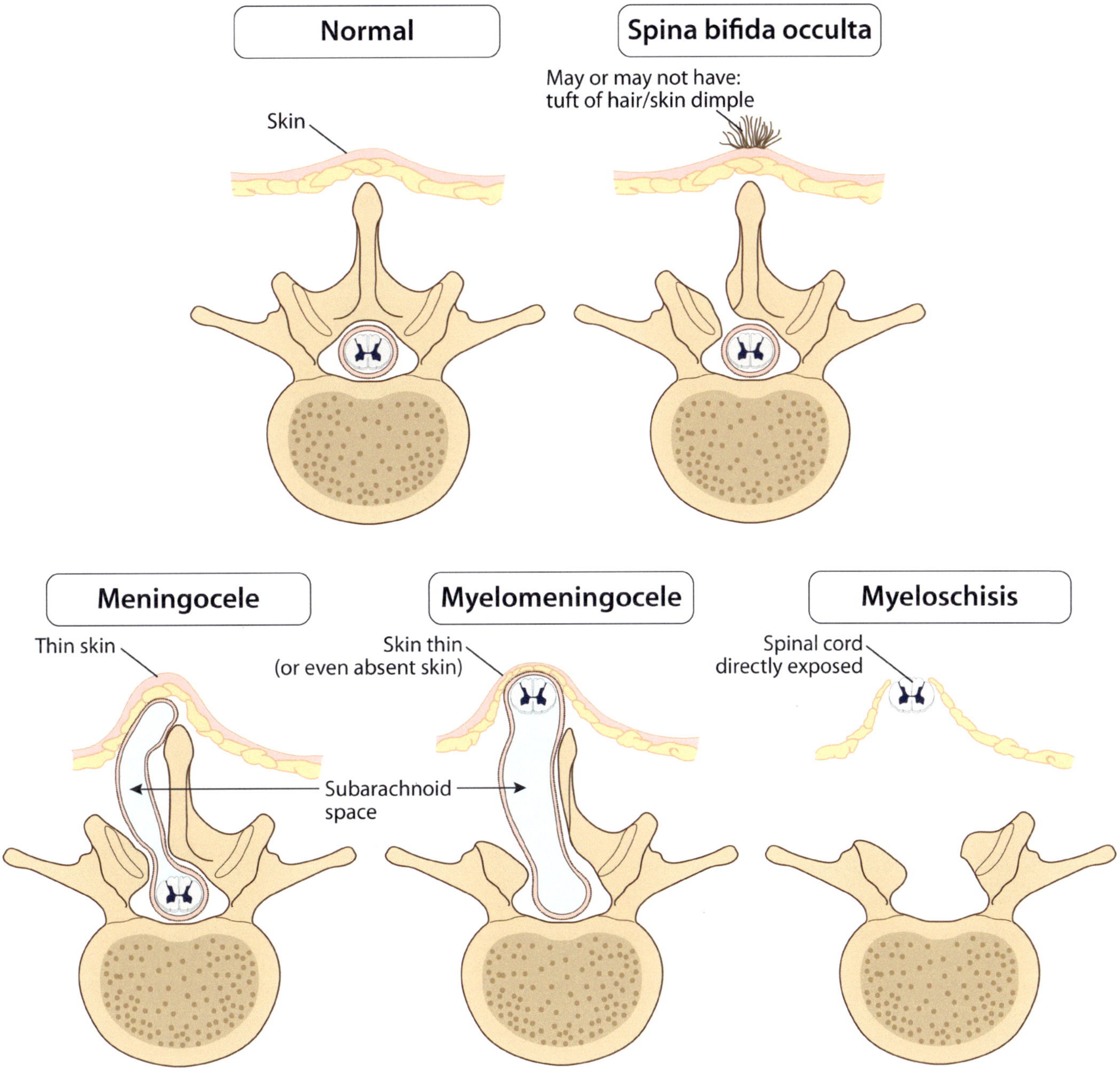

Figure 6.7.2 - Neural tube defects

IV. Neural Tube Defects

A. Caudal defects

1. Spina bifida occulta: cleft in vertebra
2. Meningocele: cleft + herniation of meninges
3. Myelomeningocele: cleft + herniation of meninges + spinal cord
4. Myeloschisis: cleft + herniation of spinal cord (no meninges or skin)

B. Cranial defect

1. Anencephaly: defect in calvaria and skin → exposed/destroyed neural tissue (not viable)

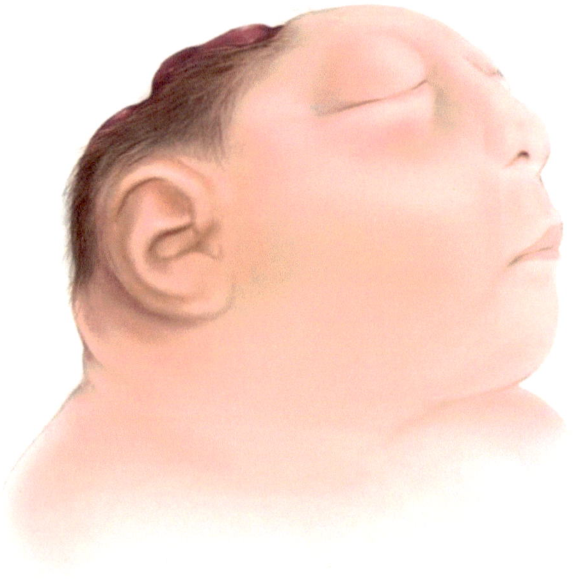

Photo Credit: Centers for Disease Control and Prevention [Public Domain]

Figure 6.7.3 - Anencephaly

V. Risk Factors
   A. Folic acid deficiency
   B. Maternal diabetes
   C. Maternal exposure to medications
      1. Valproate
      2. Carbamazepine

VI. Holoprosencephaly
   A. Embryonic forebrain fails to separate into two cerebral hemispheres
      1. Commonly associated with midline facial defects
   B. Occurs in weeks 5-6
      1. Result of mutations in sonic hedgehog signaling

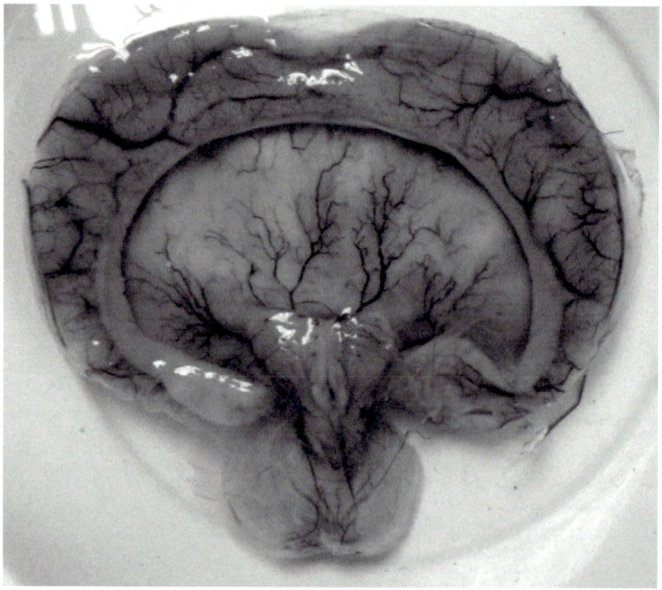

Photo Credit: Image by Stevenfruitsmaak via http://www.jmedicalcasereports.com/content/2/1/251

Figure 6.7.4 - Gross specimen of holoprosencephaly

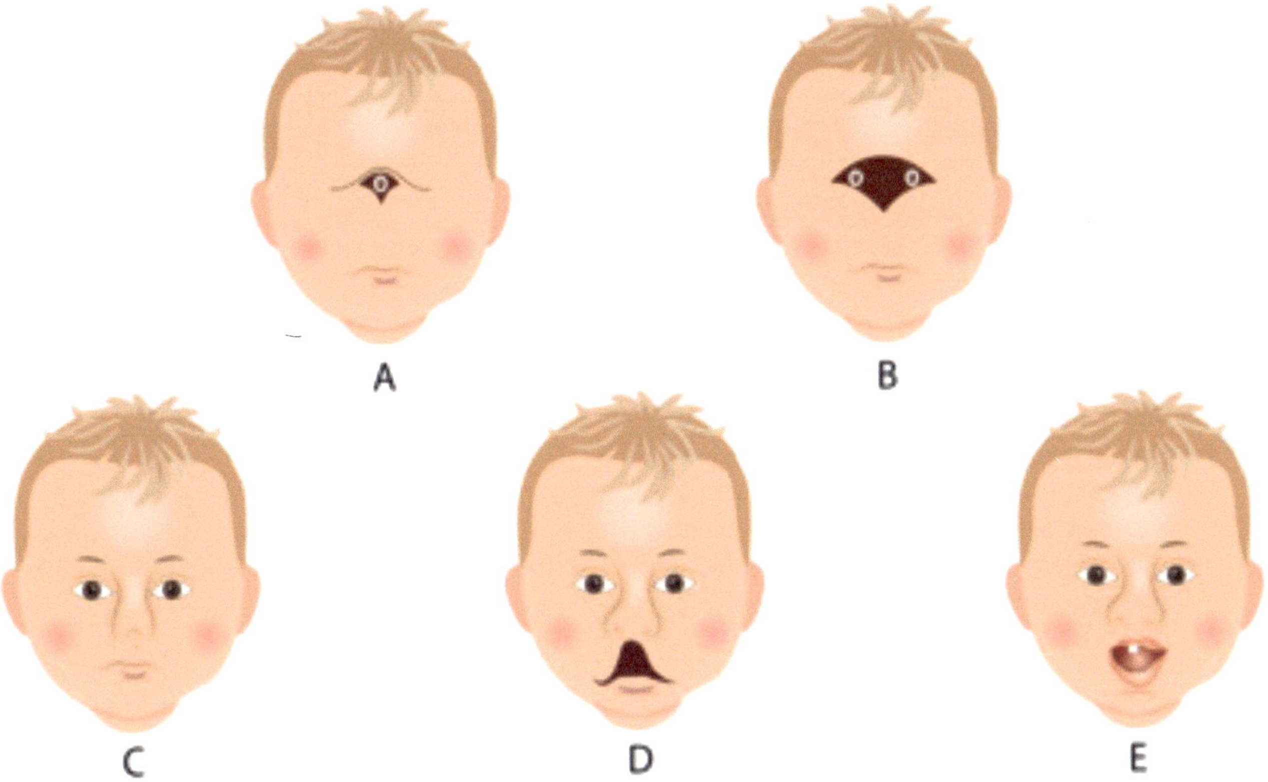

Figure 6.1.7 - Spectrum of midline defects and holoprosencephaly

VII. Lissencephaly

A. AKA "agyria" = smooth brain

B. Failure of neuronal migration during weeks 12-24

C. No gyri or sulci

D. Associated with microcephaly and ventriculomegaly

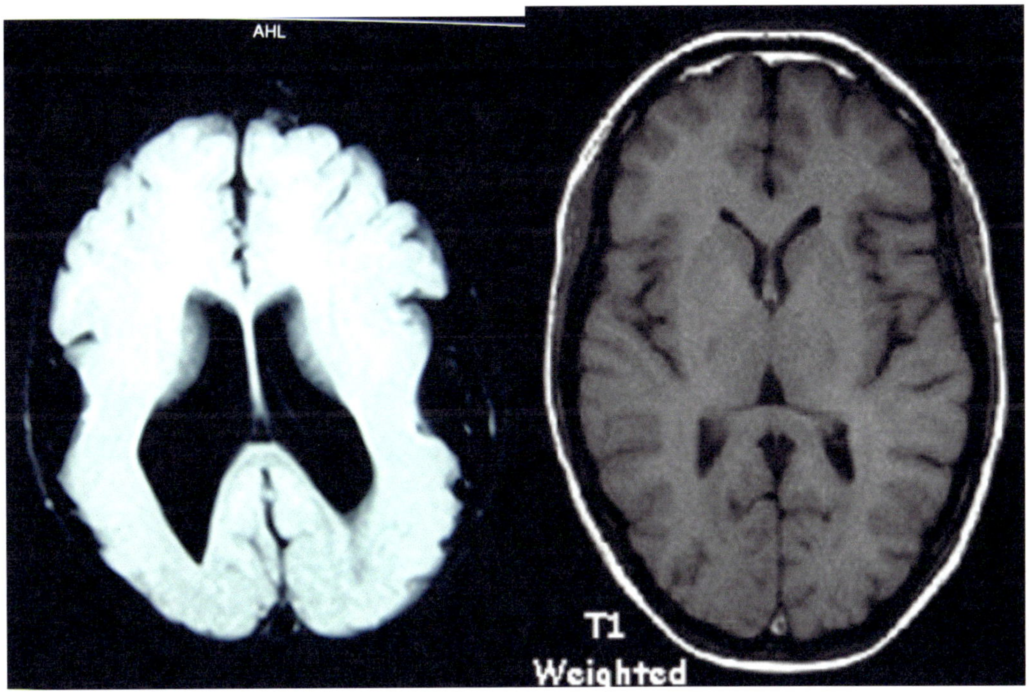

Photo Credit: (left) Ralphelg [CC BY-SA 3.0 (https://creativecommons.org/licenses/by-sa/3.0)], (right) KieranMaher at English Wikibooks [Public domain]

Figure 6.7.5 - Lissencephaly MRI (left), Normal (right)

REVIEW QUESTIONS

1. A 56-year-old man presents with a four week history of headaches, fatigue, vision problems, and erectile dysfunction. An MRI is performed and the man is diagnosed with a pituitary adenoma. What is the embryologic origin of the cells affected by the tumor?

- **Correct answer: Surface ectoderm**
- **MRI findings indicate pituitary adenoma**
- **The symptoms are more consistent with an anterior pituitary adenoma, as opposed to a posterior pituitary issue**
- **The anterior pituitary gland arises from surface ectoderm, ultimately derived from the ectoderm**

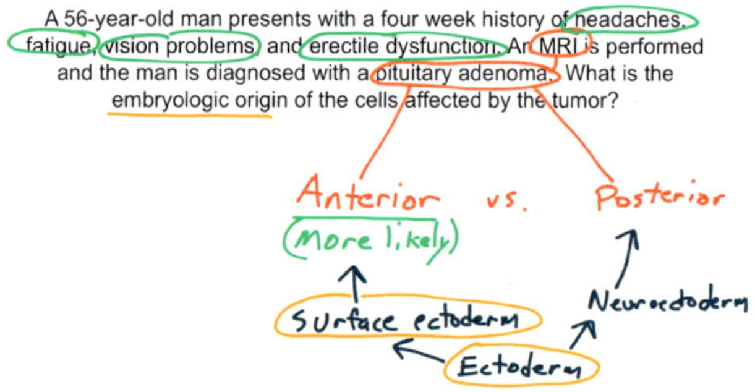
A 56-year-old man presents with a four week history of headaches, fatigue, vision problems, and erectile dysfunction. An MRI is performed and the man is diagnosed with a pituitary adenoma. What is the embryologic origin of the cells affected by the tumor?
Anterior
vs.
Posterior
(More likely)
Surface ectoderm
Neuroectoderm
Ectoderm

Section II - Posterior Fossa Malformations

I. Posterior Fossa Malformations
   A. Chiari malformation type I
   B. Chiari malformation type II
   C. Dandy-Walker malformation

II. Chiari Malformation Overview
   A. Congenital anomaly at the craniocervical junction → downward displacement of cerebellar structures

III. Chiari Type I: Definition
   A. Abnormally shaped cerebellar tonsils displaced below the foramen magnum

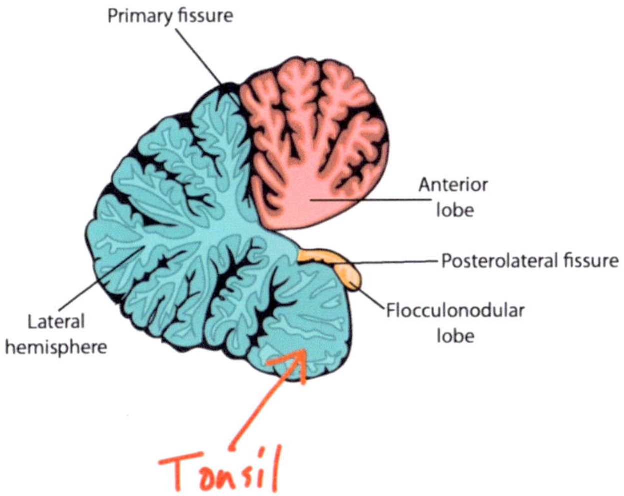

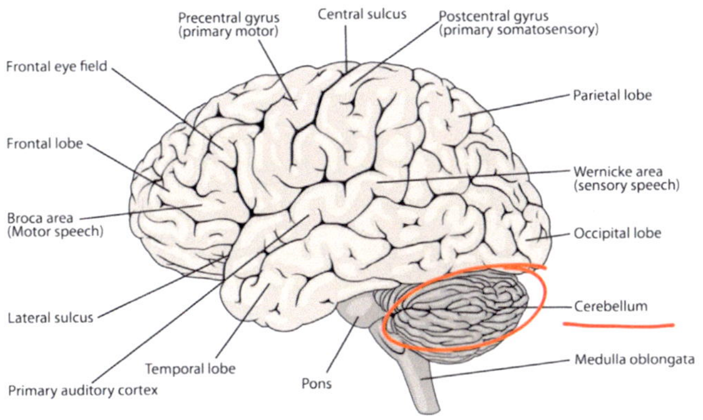

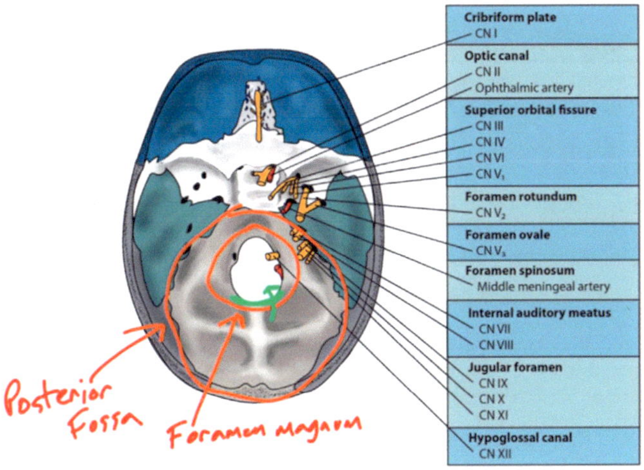

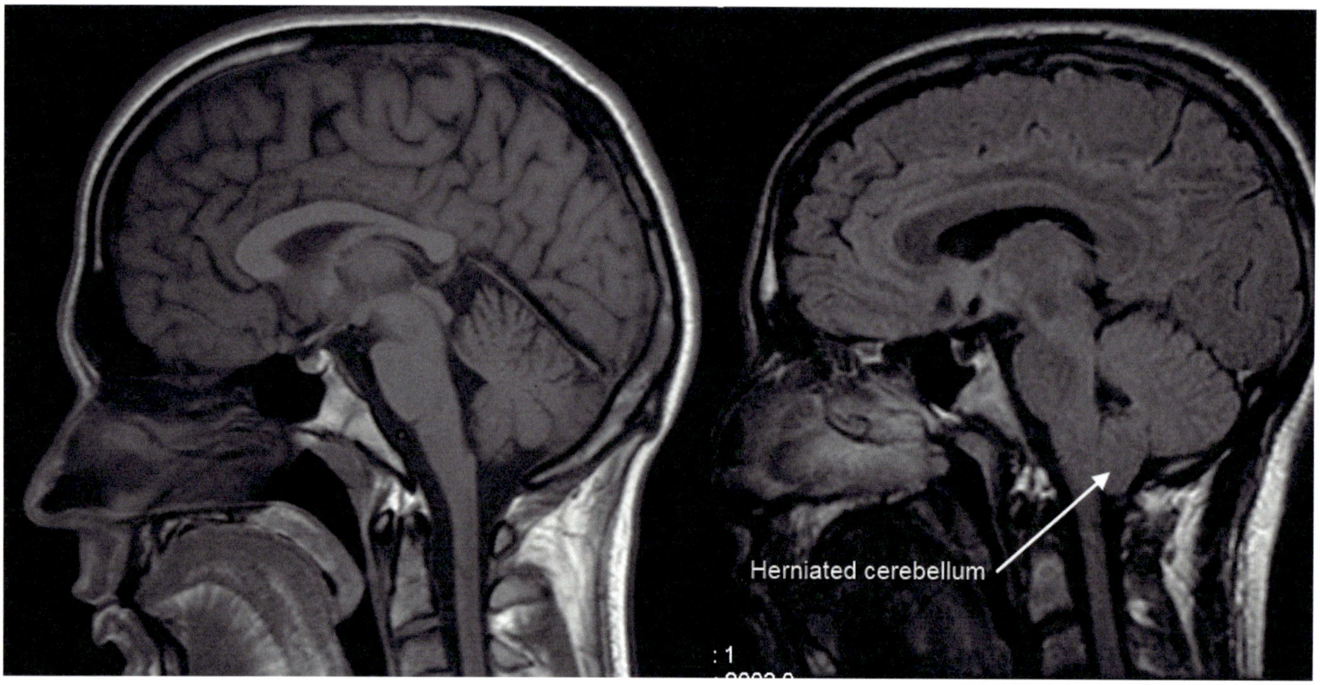

Figure 6.7.6 - Normal (left) vs Chiari type I (right) MRI

IV. Chiari Type I: Presentation

A. Usually asymptomatic until adulthood but can cause numerous issues

B. Noncommunicating hydrocephalus: ↑ ICP and papilledema

C. Meningeal irritation: head and neck pain

D. Brainstem compression: cranial neuropathies (esp. CN IX and X → problems speaking, swallowing, breathing)

E. Cerebellar dysfunction: ataxia and nystagmus

F. Syringomyelia

V. Syringomyelia

A. Fluid filled cavity of cyst called a syrinx → compresses fibers of the spinothalamic tract (pain/temp. sensation)

B. Typically occurs between C2-T9 → "cape like" distribution

C. Commonly occurs with Chiari type I and II malformations

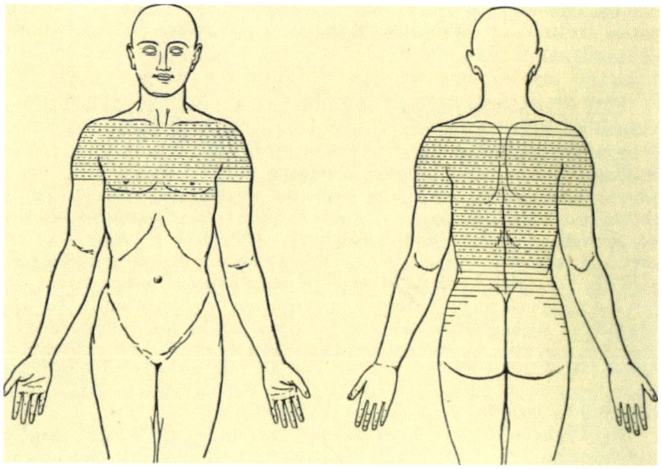

Figure 6.7.7 - Cape-like distribution of sensory loss in syringomyelia

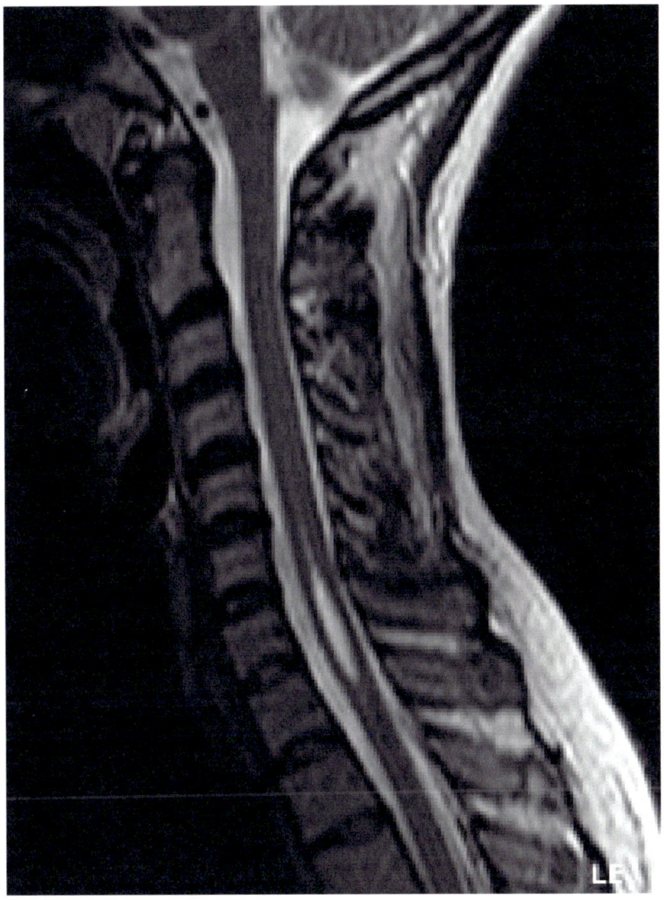

Photo Credit: Cyborg Ninja at English Wikipedia [Public domain]

Figure 6.7.8 - Lateral cervical MRI in syringomyelia

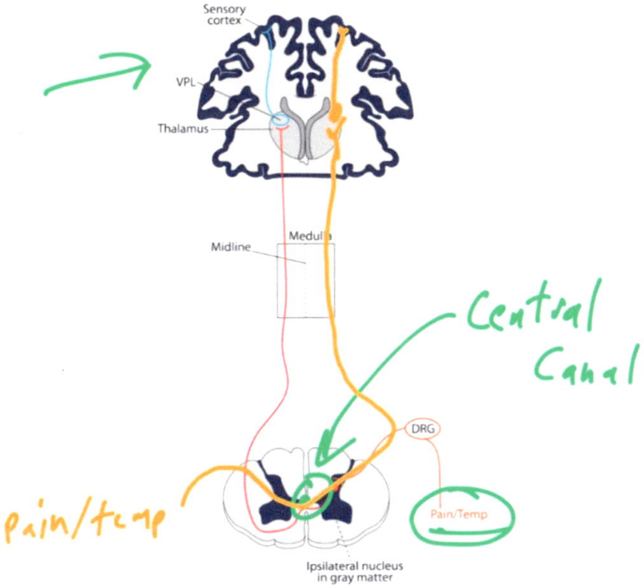

VI. Chiari Type II

A. Herniation of both the vermis and tonsils below the foramen magnum

B. Similar presentation to Chiari type I

1. More likely to present earlier and with more severe symptoms (esp. cranial neuropathies and breathing issues)

C. Very closely associated with myelomeningocele

1. Almost all myelomeningocele patients have Chiari type II

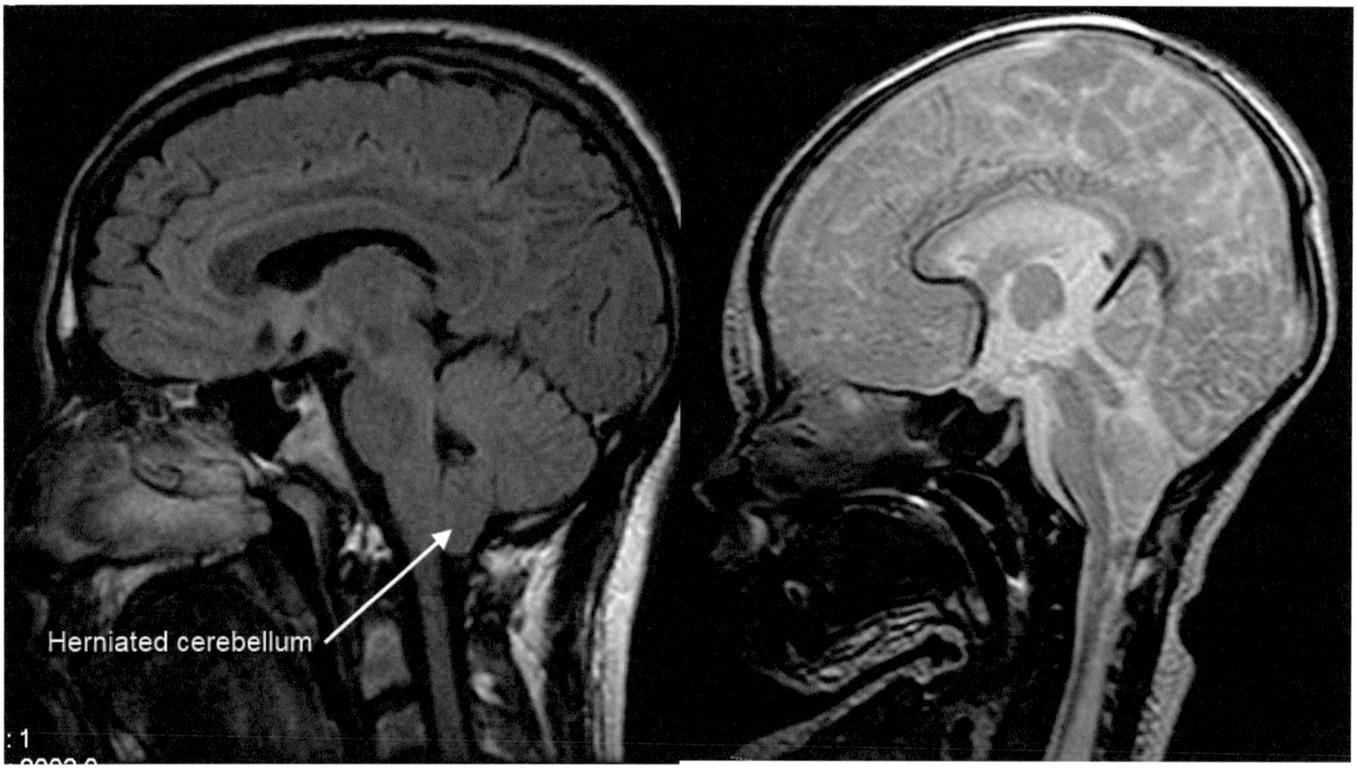

Photo Credit: Basket of Puppies [CC BY-SA 3.0 (https://creativecommons.org/licenses/by-sa/3.0)] (left); Photo by Hellerhoff via Creative Commons https://commons.wikimedia.org/wiki/File:Chiari-Malformation_MRT_T2_sag.jpg (right)

Figure 6.7.9 - Chiari type I (left) vs type II (right) MRI

VII. Dandy-Walker Malformation

A. Developmental anomaly

1. Fourth ventricle fails to close
2. Cerebellar vermis fails to develop

B. The consequence is enlargement of the 4th ventricle which fills the posterior fossa → hydrocephalus

C. Associated with many different chromosomal abnormalities, environmental exposures, and other sporadic organ defects

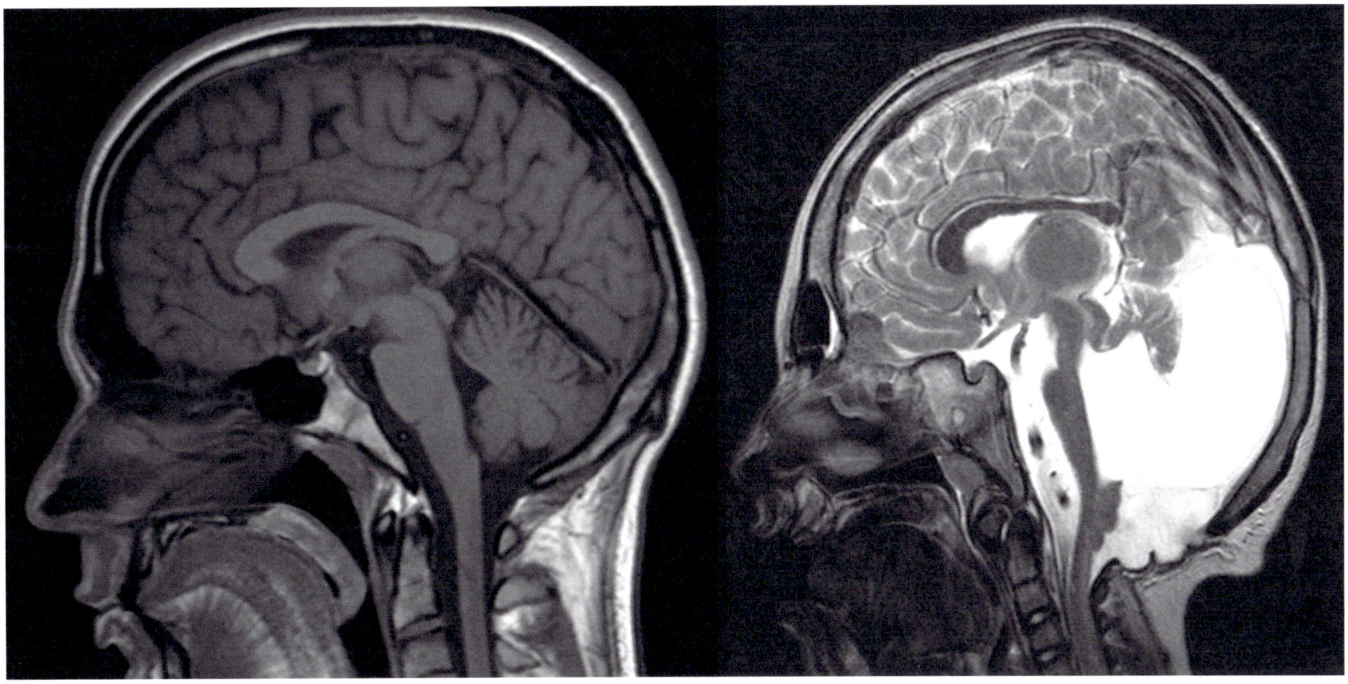

Photo Credit: Helmut Januschka [CC BY-SA 3.0 (http://creativecommons.org/licenses/by-sa/3.0/)] (left); Hellerhoff [CC BY-SA 3.0 (https://creativecommons.org/licenses/by-sa/3.0)] (right)

Figure 6.7.10 - Dandy-Walker MRI (right) vs normal (left)

REVIEW QUESTIONS

1. A newborn girl does not make any effort to breath immediately upon delivery. After respiratory intervention is implemented, imaging is performed. Results indicate a posterior fossa malformation and there is significant compression of the brainstem. The 4th ventricle appears to have developed and closed appropriately. Which posterior fossa malformation is most consistent with this presentation?

   - **Answer: Chiari type II**
   - **The posterior fossa malformation has lead to compression of the brainstem which has likely lead to neuropathy of cranial nerve 10, the vagus nerve, which is needed for initiating breathing**
   - **The malformation in this patient presented early (infant) and is severe (apnea) which makes Chiari type II malformation more likely than Chiari type I**
   - **A Dandy-Walker malformation is unlikely because imaging indicates the 4th ventricle has developed and closed appropriately**

Made in the USA
Monee, IL
03 May 2026

49398022R00069